Coleman's Laws

The Twelve Medical Truths
You Must Know To Survive

Vernon Coleman

European Medical Journal

A catalogue record for this book is available from the British Library.

The author
Vernon Coleman MB ChB DSc is a medical practitioner with many years of experience as a GP. He is the author of over 100 books, many of which are available as kindle books on Amazon. For a list of books please see Vernon Coleman's author page on Amazon. For details of the author please visit www.vernoncoleman.com

Dedication

To Donna Antoinette: brave as a lion and sensitive as a kitten.

As Antoine de Saint Exupéry might have written (if he had been a bit more of a romantic): 'Love does not consist only in gazing at each other (delightful though that may be), but also in looking outward together in the same direction.'

CONTENTS

Preface

We all want to trust our doctor. We want to believe that we can trust him or her because life is so much easier that way. We want to believe that if we fall ill there will be someone honest, honourable, intelligent, wise, caring and compassionate to whom we can turn. If things are otherwise then we would prefer not to know.

But things have changed in the last few years. Outside influences (from drug companies, politicians and lawmakers) mean that these days very few of us can trust our doctor; not, at least, in that all-trusting way people used to trust their doctors. Trusting your doctor can be hazardous to your health.

Things have changed quite rapidly.

When I first wrote my book *How To Stop Your Doctor Killing You* in the mid 1990s the book proved popular with some readers but attracted a good deal of disapproval from others. Many people acknowledged that there might be some bad doctors around but believed that most doctors were good and that *their* doctor was certainly one of the good ones. That has changed. When, in 2003, I published a second and larger edition of *How To Stop Your Doctor Killing You* readers leapt on the book with much greater enthusiasm and, it has to be said, with some apparent relief.

Today, things are getting worse at a frightening rate.

The majority of doctors and nurses seem to have forgotten why they were trained and why they are paid. Passion and purpose have disappeared as the healing professions have become part of an industry; obsessed by the need to make a profit and unconcerned with such unprofitable concepts as ethics and caring.

I suspect that all readers of this book make some effort to ensure that the tyres on their cars have plenty of tread and that their brakes are in good, working condition. Everyone knows that motorcars can kill, and so sensible individuals do what they can to protect themselves.

And yet many more people die each year as a result of medical 'accidents' than die as a result of road accidents.

Put another way, this means that your doctor is far more likely to kill you than your car. Not knowing how to protect yourself from poor medical decisions is far more dangerous than driving around in a poorly maintained motorcar.

The underlying problem is that even good, kind, conscientious doctors — doctors who are honest and honourable, who care about their work and who do their very best for their patients — can still make people ill. And can still kill.

Many (though by no means all) of the problems caused by doctors are a result of prescription drug consumption. When he writes out a prescription your doctor has to rely upon the honesty and integrity of the drug company making the product he is prescribing. And since most drug companies do not operate in an honest way that is a fundamental error of trust which can lead to many problems. You suffer from your doctor's trust in the drug company.

These days medicine is so complex, and drugs so powerful, that you don't have to be an evil doctor to be a bad doctor.

To that you must add the fact that all patients are individual and different. A drug which has proved effective and safe when given to 99 or 999 patients may still prove dangerous and deadly when given to the 100th or the 1000th patient.

Every patient who takes a drug — even a well-tried drug — is participating in an experiment. Most doctors either do not understand this or they forget it in the heat of daily practice. And, of course, prescribing drugs is just one of the things doctors do.

The bottom line is that however good your doctor is — and however much you may trust him or her — you must share the responsibility for your own health and you must know when to tell your doctor if you think that the treatment with which he or she is providing you could be causing problems.

* * *

Things aren't going to get any better. Indeed, my view is that everything will continue to get worse. Medicine is complex, and becoming ever more complex by the day. Medical students and young nurses are being taught within an environment which is geared towards defending the system and protecting drug companies. Responsibility has been separated from authority. In many hospitals patients are regarded (if they are regarded at all) as a nuisance.

Things will only change for the better when patients, and the honest professionals who do care, are prepared to stand up and make their voices heard.

Tell your friends, neighbours and colleagues what you read in this book. Share what you have learnt. Things don't have to be as bad as they are. But we are the only people who can make a difference. Reasonable men adapt themselves to the world around them. Unreasonable men try to adapt the world to themselves. So all progress depends on unreasonable men. Let us all be unreasonable.

* * *

I have built this book around twelve basic laws of medicine which I have, over the years, formulated for my own benefit, as a doctor, an author, a concerned relative and a patient. I have illustrated the twelve laws with clinical anecdotes and scientific data.

My twelve laws are designed to help you make sure that you get the best out of your doctor (and every other doctor who treats you) — and to minimise your chances of being made ill by a doctor.

Vernon Coleman August 2006

Author's Boring But Important Notes

1. This book is not intended to be, and cannot be, an alternative to personal, professional medical advice. Readers should immediately consult a trained and properly qualified health professional, whom they trust and respect, for advice about any symptom or health problem which requires diagnosis, treatment or any kind of medical attention. Readers should always consult a qualified doctor before changing or stopping medication, before changing their diet or before beginning any exercise programme. While the advice and information in this book are believed to be accurate at the time of writing, neither the author nor the publisher can accept any legal responsibility or liability for errors or omissions which may have been made.

2. Many authors of medical books try to make themselves (and their books) look well-informed by padding out their work with pages and pages of references. My books do not contain scientific references. There is a very good reason for this. If I listed all the references I've used in researching and writing this book the reference section would be as long as the text, there would be twice as many pages and the book would cost twice as much to print and distribute. My guarantee that the material in this book is well-founded is built upon my credibility as an author. If my readers find that I've made stuff up, or made mistakes, then no one will buy my next book. This is what I do for a living and it's in my professional and financial interest to make sure it's accurate.

Vernon Coleman 2006

Coleman's 1st Law Of Medicine

If you are receiving treatment for an existing disease and you develop new symptoms then, until proved otherwise, you should assume that the new symptoms are caused by the treatment you are receiving.

1

Doctors are notoriously reluctant to admit that the treatments they recommend can do harm. There are several reasons for this. First, they often simply don't know how dangerous drugs can be (doctors rarely bother to read drug company information sheets). Second, they are frightened of being sued. (Doctors fear that if they admit that their treatment made someone ill they will receive a letter from a lawyer.) And finally, there is a natural human unwillingness to admit responsibility for something that has gone wrong. This brand of unwillingness is unusually well-developed among doctors who are encouraged to think of themselves as godlike by many of their other more passive patients. Admitting to having made someone ill reminds doctors that they are mortal and fallible.

Because doctors almost never admit that the drugs they have prescribed might have caused unpleasant or dangerous side effects, very few incidences of drug-induced illness are reported to the official watchdogs which exist to measure and assess drug side effects. This enables doctors and drug companies to claim that prescription drugs are safe. (The word 'safe' is, of course, relative. Even though the number of reported side effects is absurdly low, doctors are now officially one of the top four causes of death and serious injury in the world. They share the top four spots with cancer, heart disease and stroke.)

2

Side effects are far commoner than most people (including doctors) think. Four out of every ten patients who take a prescription drug will develop side effects. Some side effects will be mild and others will be unpleasant but many will be dangerous and potentially life-threatening.

3

Drug side effects can (and usually do) cause problems when you least expect them. None of us is immune. And both doctors and patients are usually far too slow to consider drug side effects when they are looking for a cause for new symptoms. We are all likely to forget or under-estimate the danger.

After I damaged my shoulder joint (don't ask how — you don't want to know and wouldn't believe it) I started taking soluble aspirin to reduce the inflammation.

On a trip to France I started using a local variety of soluble aspirin. It dissolved much more speedily than the English variety.

My shoulder was improving nicely.

But then I developed another, quite separate problem. I started getting severe muscle pain in my left calf.

Donna Antoinette, my wife, asked if it could be due to the aspirin. I dismissed her fears. I was taking only a small dose of aspirin — and had been taking the same dose for some time without trouble.

Because the pain had started while I was walking my first fear was that it was intermittent claudication — indicative of a blocked artery in my leg. But my pulse was good so I wondered if I could have a deep vein thrombosis. It seemed extremely unlikely since aspirin is a good anti-clotting drug. I compared my painful calf with my other one using my tie as a substitute for the tape measure I didn't have. The painful calf wasn't swollen. Besides, the pain was too much like a cramp. (Being a doctor can be a bit of a nuisance at times.)

That night I hardly slept. I was close to calling for an ambulance.

What could cause such severe muscle cramps?

And then it occurred to me that a metabolic alkalosis is another possible cause of cramps.

Why could I be suffering from a sudden alkalosis?

My wife was still quietly and politely wondering about the aspirin.

I checked the packet. And discovered that in addition to the aspirin the tablets contained sodium bicarbonate. The bicarbonate was there to help the tablets dissolve quickly. And even though I was on a low dose there was enough sodium bicarbonate to cause the alkalosis. And the cramps.

I stopped the aspirin. And a day later the cramps disappeared. This embarrassing story reinforces Coleman's 1st Law of Medicine which states that if you have a health problem which requires treatment and you acquire new symptoms then the new symptoms are probably caused by the treatment you're taking.

Side effects are a major cause of illness today. And it isn't just the main constituent of a drug which can cause problems.

4

According to the *Journal of the American Medical Association:* 'Adverse drug reactions are the fourth leading cause of death in America. Reactions to prescription and over-the-counter medications kill far more people annually than all illegal drug use combined.'

5

The incidence of drug side effects would not matter so much if all prescriptions were necessary and life-saving. But they aren't. On the contrary most prescriptions are unnecessary.

6

There are hugely profitable prescription drugs on the market which have saved no lives at all but which have killed ten times as many people as the attack which took place in America on 11th September 2001.

7

The power of the drug companies is vast.

In America the drug industry is represented by over 1,200 full time political lobbyists — including 40 former members of Congress. Drug companies contribute millions to federal election campaigns and spend over $12 billion a year handing out drug samples and employing drug pushers (known as sales representatives) to influence doctors to prescribe specifically branded drugs.

In just about every Westernised country in the world doctors receive most of their official (and, therefore, theoretically independent) post graduate education through meetings (sponsored by drug companies) and journals (which rely heavily on drug company advertising).

You will not be surprised to read that drug companies do not spend a good deal of time or effort warning doctors about drug side effects.

8

The drug industry does not exist to find or make cures or treatments for people. It does not exist to help people. It does not exist to save lives. It exists solely to make money. Doctors must know this. But as a profession they are, nevertheless, married to the industry and their actions suggest that many doctors regard their primary loyalty as being to the drug industry rather than to their patients. Doctors are encouraged to be loyal to the pharmaceutical industry by governments which consistently bow to drug company demands.

It comes as a shock to some people to realise that drug companies (like food companies and supermarkets) exist to make money. (These days they exist to make it for the executives who run the companies rather than the shareholders who own them but that's another story). No large business exists to please the customers except in that it wants to encourage customers to keep buying its products. And drug companies, whose customers are largely captive, don't have to worry about that. Indeed, one of the main problems with drug companies is that the real customers for their products — patients — are removed from the decision-making processes which lead to a rise or fall in corporate profits.

Drug company executives are beholden to the short-term share price of their company. They must work constantly to defend the share price in order to defend their own bonuses and share options.

As I explained in previous books (notably *Toxic Stress* and *Animal Rights Human Wrongs)* our world is now controlled not by the needs of individuals but by the needs of corporations. And naturally corporations (and institutions, associations and governments) are not restrained by ethical considerations.

Drug companies don't have hearts or consciences. They want to sell you drugs. The company doesn't give a fig whether the drug makes you ill or kills you. The company just wants your money.

9

In response to a newspaper article discussing whether or not doctors can judge the claims made by drug company representatives one reader wrote: I suspect that the training that a medical practitioner receives both before and after qualifying equips him or her to judge the quality of information received and reliability of the source. Otherwise what has been achieved by a lengthy and continuing education?'

I'm afraid I have bad news for this trusting patient.

Most doctors in practice today learned next to nothing about drugs while at medical school. When I qualified as a doctor my knowledge of practical prescribing was pitiful. And after qualification most of the training a doctor receives is paid for by drug companies.

Drug company representatives are trained to know all there is to know about one or two particular drugs.

(Many such representatives seem to learn the information by rote. When I was a general practitioner I discovered that if I stopped a rep in mid flow he or she would invariably have to go back to the beginning and start all over again.)

It is safest to assume that most doctors know little about the drugs they prescribe; and that the little they know they learn from the companies that make those drugs.

10

If given a choice between an old treatment and a new treatment you should always choose the old treatment.

New drugs are more dangerous than old ones. Drug side effects only appear after time. The big advantage of a drug that has been around for years is that it is unlikely to be the world's most dangerous drug. The longer a treatment has been around the more will be known about it. You should only take a new and untested drug when you have tried all the old and tested drugs and they haven't worked.

11

Many huge-selling drugs are launched on the basis of trials involving relatively few people. So, for example, consider a trial which involves 100 patients. If just one in 1,000 people who take the drug dies from it the chances are high that the trial of 100 patients will show nothing amiss. But if the drug is then assumed to be safe and prescribed for 10,000,000 people worldwide (a highly likely occurrence) it means that 10,000 people will die as a result of taking the drug.

This sort of carnage is probably acceptable if the drug is life-saving and is only prescribed for patients who might otherwise die.

But if the drug is prescribed for something which is not life-threatening (such as hayfever) then all those deaths are entirely unnecessary.

12

Everyone is different. A pill which saves your life may kill your next door neighbour.

13

A 13-year-old child weighing 6 stone will probably receive the same dose of medication as a 45-year-old man weighing 20 stone.

The same medicines (often in the same doses) are prescribed for young and old, male and female, fat and thin.

This is bizarre, illogical and indefensible.

No one bothers to do any research into how much of a drug should be given to which type of patient. Why should they? The vast majority of drug research is done by, or on behalf of, drug companies. Adjusting doses to suit particular patients is of no interest to them. All they want to do is sell drugs.

And so everyone (young or old, small or big) gets the biggest dose the drug company can sell.

14

Never take a new drug if you are alone in the house. If you are alone and you have an anaphylactic shock reaction you could die. Anaphylactic shock reactions are commoner than most people imagine. The number of people suffering from potentially life-threatening allergic reactions has increased by more than 300% in a decade and, for example, in one recent year around 30,000 people in the United Kingdom (UK) had anaphylactic shock reactions). Anaphylactic shock reactions can — and do — kill. If there is someone else with you there will be someone able to ring for a doctor and an ambulance.

15

In medicine the word 'new' when used to describe a drug means two things: the drug is expensive and no one yet knows whether it will cure you or kill you.

16

More and more prescription drugs are being made available 'over the counter' without a prescription. Every year another clump of potentially lethal drugs is licensed for patients to buy without any medical advice.

This is, of course, incredibly dangerous. It is reckless of pharmacies to sell such dangerous drugs and it is reckless of governments to allow them to do so.

But it happens because it suits everyone in the medicine business.

Drug companies want drugs to be made available over the counter because this enables them to advertise their drugs more freely, to sell more of them and to make much bigger profits.

Governments want drugs to be available over the counter because this means that patients have to pay and the Government doesn't.

Doctors are enthusiastic about patients buying their own drugs because it cuts down their workload and gives them more time to fill in forms.

And pharmacists are keen on selling drugs over the counter because it helps boost their profits.

The only people who lose out are patients.

This policy means that patients have more responsibility forced on them and are likely to die or become seriously ill if they make an error of any kind in making a diagnosis or choosing a treatment.

17

High street shoppers are now encouraged to purchase cholesterol lowering drugs even though (as I first revealed in my book *How to Stop Your Doctor Killing You* in 1996) there is really no clear evidence proving that these drugs are both safe and necessary. Your friendly local pharmacist will sell you a test to find out if you have too much cholesterol and then, if you have, sell you just the drug to deal with it.

In April 2005, the *Drug and Therapeutics Bulletin* revealed that the British Government had re-classified the cholesterol lowering drug Simvastatin as an over-the-counter product, called Zocor Heart-Pro, available to be purchased without a prescription, although this decision was 'not based on robust evidence of clinical benefit.

The *Drug and Therapeutics Bulletin* claimed that it had uncovered evidence that the medicines regulator (the Medicines and Healthcare products Regulatory Agency — MHRA) had inaccurately reported the consultation which preceded the re-classification. In November 2003, the MHRA had published a consultation document on the proposed re-classification of this drug. One hundred responses were received from a wide range of professional organisations, patient groups and individuals. The MHRA announced that about two thirds of respondents were in favour of the proposal. Not true, according to the *Drug and Therapeutics Bulletin.*

'...our analysis of the 80 responses that the MHRA has made available for public scrutiny indicates that 31% of these respondents offered at least some support for the re-classification, 35% clearly opposed it and the rest offered no clear opinion either way...Even if all 20 of the withheld responses are assumed to have been in favour of the re-classification, only 45% of all respondents at most could be described as supporting the proposal.

So, to put it politely, the MHRA had bent the truth.

Why would it do this?

Three reasons.

First, drug companies can make far more money when a drug is made available without prescription. They can sell their product to far more people and don't have to worry about persuading doctors to prescribe it.

Second, the Government saves money because all the patients who take the drug have to pay for it themselves. In the UK around 1.8 million people were taking statins when the drug was first made available without a prescription. The cost to the NHS was £700 million and rising fast. With drug company campaigns to persuade doctors to prescribe the drugs proving extremely effective it was estimated that the NHS bill would exceed £2 billion a year within a few years.

Thirdly, many of the people associated with the MHRA are alleged to have long-standing links with the drug industry. Some own shares in drug companies.

I have been writing about such matters since 1970 and so I wasn't in the slightest bit surprised to hear that once again a Government agency had acted in a way designed to benefit a drug company and to put ordinary citizens at risk.

The *Drug and Therapeutics Bulletin* reported that no trials had assessed the drug's long-term effectiveness in its target group — people likely to be at moderate risk of having a heart attack.

'The lack of such research,' said the *Drug and Therapeutics Bulletin,* 'raises serious questions about whether people are unknowingly wasting their money — around £170 a year — on a treatment that might not work. Also, crucially, since people can be sold Zocor Heart-Pro without a detailed assessment that includes measurement of blood pressure and cholesterol levels, some could be wrongly classed and treated as being at only moderate risk of a heart attack, when in reality their risk is very much higher.'

Consumers finding a drug freely available without prescription would, of course, not be aware of the nature and extent of the problems associated with drugs of this type.

When NASA astronaut Dr Duane Graveline had a heart attack he was given a statin to reduce the risk of a recurrence. Six weeks after starting the drug he lost some of his memory for six hours. The loss was so severe that he did not recognise either his wife or his own home. On recovering, Dr Graveline took himself off the drug but, a year later, decided to try it again. He had another attack of what is known as 'transient global amnesia' (TGA) which wiped out every memory since early childhood. This attack lasted twelve hours. There are hundreds of examples of statins causing TGA. Quite apart from the fears and anxieties these attacks produce it is scary to think of the consequences if a surgeon or a bus driver had one of these attacks.

Amnesia isn't the only problem linked to these drugs. One study found a 25% increase in newly diagnosed cancer among older people after four years treatment with a statin. The cancers which seem most likely to develop include cancer of the breast and cancer of the gastrointestinal tract.

Other side effects include congestive heart failure, neurological damage, extreme fatigue, nausea, muscle weakness, gastrointestinal problems and pain.

18

Doctors have no idea how long to give drugs for. When prescribing antibiotics, for example, one doctor will hand out a prescription for five days, a second will write a prescription for seven days, a third will dispense a ten day supply and a fourth will give a prescription for fourteen days. All for the same patient with the same symptoms.

Only the most bigoted member of the medical establishment would dare to describe medicine as a science.

19

A friend of mine had labyrinthitis for which his doctor prescribed a drug called prochlorperazine. Within hours my friend had developed bad dizziness when sitting up and a new symptom: ataxia. (He had difficulty in controlling body movements.) He telephoned the doctor and reported what had happened. The doctor immediately changed his diagnosis and told my friend that he might have a brain tumour. He increased the dose of the prochlorperazine and said he would arrange for a brain scan to be performed. When the dizziness and the ataxia got worse my friend's wife telephoned me to tell me what was happening. She was, not surprisingly, in tears.

'He's on prochlorperazine?' I asked.

'Yes,' she whispered. 'But it doesn't seem to be helping.'

'Stop it,' I told her. 'Stop the prochlorperazine and I think he'll be better.'

They stopped the prochlorperazine.

The dizziness on sitting up and the ataxia were gone within hours.

Both symptoms are. possible side effects of prochlorperazine.

20

Here's another true story about drug side effects. It involves a reader of mine.

My reader (an elderly man) went to his local surgery complaining of breathlessness.

A nurse gave him a spirometer to blow into. (A spirometer is a simple instrument which measures lung function). My reader huffed and puffed but could not do much with it. So on the basis of this single test the nurse diagnosed a wonderful new disease called Chronic Obstructive Airways Disease (COPD). (Making this diagnosis was a pretty stupid (not to say dangerous) thing to do. If my reader had put his hands around the nurse's throat she would have not been able to blow into the tube either. But it wouldn't prove she had COPD.)

'You have a chronic cough and bring up sputum every day, don't you?' she said.

'No,' he replied.

'Oh well, never mind,' she replied. 'I'll put you down as suffering from chronic obstructive pulmonary disease anyway.'

My reader had no other signs or symptoms of COPD. His medical history did not suggest that he was a likely candidate. But satisfied with her diagnosis the nurse then exercised her newly acquired right to prescribe and prescribed a steroid spray. Steroids are, of course, enormously powerful and equally dangerous. They should only be prescribed when absolutely essential.

Since my reader didn't have COPD the steroid spray didn't work. So the nurse gave him a spray containing both a steroid and another chemical. Since the diagnosis was wrong this did not work either.

My reader then went back to the nurse (maybe doctors are too busy attending meetings to see patients these days) and told her that the medicine she'd prescribed wasn't working. Believing in her diagnosis he trustingly asked if he could double it. The nurse, seemingly as ignorant as my reader, duly doubled the dose.

When my reader developed atrial fibrillation (a known side effect of the deadly mixture he had been given) the doctor found a gap between all his meetings and prescribed digoxin to control the fibrillation. (It did not occur to the doctor to stop the drug causing the fibrillation; possibly because he didn't know that the drug could cause fibrillation.)

Unfortunately, the digoxin slowed my reader's heartbeat so much that he started getting chest pains. So the doctor, probably fearing that the digoxin might slow the circulation, create a blood clot and cause a heart attack, started my reader on warfarin to stop his blood clotting.

My reader's breathing problem was still no better so he then had an X-ray which showed that a fall he'd had some weeks earlier had resulted in several crushed ribs. The radiologist also noticed that my reader had tuberculosis scars on his lungs.

My reader, however, was now taking steroids, digoxin and warfarin (three of the most potent goodies in the drugs business) and was considerably worse than he had been when he'd first visited the nurse.

Naturally, the doctors involved refused to accept that the drug he'd been given could have caused the atrial fibrillation. They claimed that the fact that the fibrillation had started so soon after the drug had been prescribed was just a coincidence. In truth no one could say for certain whether or not the drug had caused the heart problem but since the drug company had admitted that their product could cause problems of this type it seemed to me that to dismiss the possibility of the link was something an ostrich might have done. It was rather akin to arguing that if a man who was hit on the head with a hammer subsequently developed a headache there was no connection between the two, or that if a man got a broken arm after falling down stairs the break was merely a coincidence.

Doctors who have prescribed drugs which have caused serious side effects rarely admit that there could be a link between a drug they have prescribed and a worsening of the patient's condition. Doctors prefer almost any solution other than the awful one that a patient has been made ill by a side effect, because that means it was their fault (with all the legal and moral overtones that carries).

21

Aspirin is one of the safest and most tested drugs in the world but it is also out of patent and very cheap to make and to buy. So wonderfully idiotic rules have been introduced in many countries making it impossible to buy aspirin in anything other than very small quantities. So, for example, if you want to buy aspirin to treat your arthritis you may find that you can only buy tablets in packs of twelve. This means that the average arthritis sufferer will have to visit the chemist almost daily. Inevitably, they don't. They visit their doctor and are given a prescription for something which is almost certainly far more expensive and probably much more dangerous.

22

When a patient is given a prescription drug there is a risk that the drug will cause a side effect. When a patient is given two drugs both can, of course, cause side effects. But there is another (usually underestimated) problem. Many drugs do not interact well. If you take two drugs then your chances of developing unpleasant or lethal side effects are far greater than the chances of developing unpleasant or lethal side effects with the two individual drugs.

Taking two prescription drugs is a bit like mixing brandy and red wine. Taking three is like mixing brandy, red wine and champagne.

Drug companies, which sometimes seem to me to thrive on creating illness, often make things worse by manufacturing compound drugs which actually contain two or more drugs in one tablet or capsule. The only advantage of this is that it enables them to make many people ill. And, of course, people who are ill are usually given yet more tablets.

23

Most of the clinical research published in medical journals (and used as the basis for medical practice) is (how shall I put it to be tactful) as bent as a paperclip. Authors of clinical research articles are supposed to admit to any links they have with drug companies if those links might have a direct effect on their credibility. But general links don't count which is just as well since the vast majority of medical researchers have, at some stage in their careers, taken drug company money.

Between two thirds and three quarters of the drug trials published in major medical journals are funded by drug companies. Research conducted by drug companies which shows that a drug doesn't work or is dangerous is routinely suppressed.

Sceptics about the independence of studies funded by drug companies point to the fact that research programmes paid for by drug companies are four times as likely to produce results which are favourable to the company than are studies funded from other sources. What an amazingly useful coincidence that is.

Drug companies use a number of tricks to ensure that they get the results they want. Here are some:

* The company compares its own product with a treatment which is known to be inferior. One of the oldest tricks in the book is to compare a new painkiller or arthritis treatment with ordinary non-soluble aspirin. Since non-soluble aspirin is known to cause gastrointestinal problems it isn't easy to show that the new product is 'best'.

* The company ensures that its new wonder drug is compared either with a very low dose of the competing drug (in which case the competing drug probably doesn't work) or with a very high dose of the competing drug (in which case the competing drug probably produces very unpleasant side effects).

* One of the favourite tricks is to perform experiments on animals. These are a guaranteed success. If animals do not die or fall ill when given a drug then the company making it will announce that the drug has been proved to be safe. On the other hand, if animals do die or fall ill the company making the drug will announce that it is ignoring the results because animals are different to people. You will doubtless suspect that I am making this up. I am not. Doctors, politicians and official custodians of patient safety all accept this nonsense. (There is evidence proving this point in my book *Animal Experiments: Simple Truths* and on www.vernoncoleman.com and www.vernoncoleman.co.uk. For example, *Animal Experiments: Simple Truths* contains a list of 46 drugs which may cause tumours or cancer when given to animals but which are marketed and passed as safe for humans.)

* The company takes a lot of measurements, ignores the ones which are inconvenient and publishes the ones which make their product look good. (So, for example, they may give their product to patients for a month. At the end of the month all the patients may be dead. They will ignore that inconvenient result. But they will publish the results which show that patients had fewer symptoms after five days.)

* The company will pay numerous sets of researchers to conduct the same research. They will then ignore the results which are inconvenient and publish the one which makes their product look good.

* Drug companies will pay researchers not to publish unfavourable research results.

* At least half of the articles on drug efficacy which appear in medical journals are ghost-written by people working for drug companies. Allegedly distinguished doctors from allegedly prestigious universities then allow their names to be put on the papers — often without ever looking at the original data. The doctors do this because an academic's status depends very much on the number of scientific papers he publishes.

24

There are 348,461 clinical research papers published every week. Most of them are of no value to anyone except the author (and perhaps a drug company). Any useful ones are lost among the self-serving, useless, irrelevant, commercially-inspired dross. How can any doctor possibly be expected to read 348,461 clinical research papers every week?

25

How do medical journals make their money?

Several ways.

When an article is published in a medical journal the drug company may pay huge amounts of money to buy reprints to distribute to doctors. It is not unknown for a drug company to spend more than a million dollars buying reprints of an article.

Some medical journals charge money for an article to appear on their pages. (Normally journals and magazines pay their contributors. With some medical journals things are the other way round.)

Finally medical journals accept huge amounts of drug company advertising.

26

Statutory organisations which were founded to protect patients from badly tested or unsafe drugs are now so controlled by the drug industry that, in practice, they simply protect the interests of the pharmaceutical industry. They do this because that is the way they are structured and because most of the so-called experts who act as committee members or consultants are also receiving money from the drug companies they are supposed to be monitoring.

27

A few years ago doctors, drug companies and cancer charities were enthusiastically promoting tamoxifen as a drug that would cure and prevent breast cancer. Some advocates wanted every adult woman to take the drug every day for life. You could almost see them salivating at the thought of all those cash registers clinking away as the money poured in from around the world.

It was only when I pointed out (in my book *How To Stop Your Doctor Killing You*) that tamoxifen causes cancer of the uterus *(causes* you will note) that the drug's advocates became a little quieter in their enthusiasm for this deeply unpleasant drug.

Incidentally, tamoxifen causes liver tumours when given to rats and gonadal tumours when given to mice. Naturally, the drug's many supporters ignored this research on the grounds that animals are different to people.

28

How many parents (or, indeed, doctors) know that 90% of the medication given to newborn babies has only ever been tested on adults? Not many, I suspect. But it's true. There is evidence now that children's bodies (as well as being smaller) actually break down drugs differently to adults. This too must increase children's chances of developing serious side effects.

Two thirds of children treated in hospital are given drugs that have never been tested for use among people who are under 18 years old. Doctors have, for decades, had to guess the right dose because many drugs have never been clinically tested on children.

Similarly, drugs are not usually tested on people over 65. And so when older patients are given drugs the doctor has little idea of what may, or may not, happen.

'All this uncertainty is what makes the practice of medicine so exciting', said one particularly cruel doctor I once met.

29

In 1988, the British Government led the way internationally by issuing warnings about benzodiazepine drugs (widely used as tranquillisers and sleeping tablets and things to give to patients whose symptoms weren't easy to diagnose) and advising doctors not to prescribe them for more than two weeks at a time. (The Minister of Health at the time admitted, in a House of Commons statement, that the advice had been given as a direct result of my columns and book on the subject.) The Government recognised that the drugs could be dangerously addictive.

And yet, nearly twenty years later, it was announced that doctors were still writing out millions of prescriptions for these drugs. And, as if that wasn't bad enough, in thousands of nursing homes and hospitals nurses were handing the drugs out to elderly patients without a doctor's prescription and without the patients knowing that they were being drugged.

Around 80% of the prescriptions for sleeping tablets are for older patients who often stay on such medication for years and who suffer more than most patients from the side effects. In November 2005, I sat open mouthed with disbelief when I read an article headlined 'Sleeping pills may be doing you harm'.

'The debilitating side effects of medicines commonly prescribed for insomnia in older patients outweigh the benefits in most cases, it is claimed,' continued the news story, reporting an analysis of yet another study showing the danger associated with these drugs. A spokeswoman for a charity for the elderly said that the study was vital as there had not been enough research into the problem. (If they'd asked me I could have sent them articles and papers of mine dating back over 30 years. We need more research into the benzodiazepines like we need more lawyers.)

I have listed the horrendous side effects associated with drugs such as benzodiazepines in previous books such as *Life Without Tranquillisers* (published in 1985) and in articles I wrote from the early 1970s onwards, but it is, perhaps, enough to point out that in addition to being more addictive than heroin (or, indeed, any other illegal drug) benzodiazepine tranquillisers and sleeping tablets can cause memory and concentration problems and can result in accidents.

I am pained and ashamed to have to report that over thirty years after I first published evidence condemning the widespread use of tranquillisers and sleeping tablets, hundreds of thousands of people over 65 are still effectively being deprived of the final years of their lives because of the incompetence and stupidity of doctors and nurses.

30

Here are six pieces of research no one ever does.

1. Do drugs act differently when given to men and women? How do drugs act differently when given to elderly patients or to children?

2. When prescribed for a routine infection should antibiotics be given for three days, five days, seven days, ten days, fourteen days or what?

3. In which patients are non-drug therapies more effective than drugs?

4. Most of the drugs on the market are merely variations on a relatively small number of themes. So, for example, there are scores of different antibiotics available and scores of different painkillers on the market. But many of these are identical — differing only in that they are made by different drug companies. When will someone compare the effectiveness and safety of these different drugs?

5. We are aware that many drugs interact badly. If your doctor gives you drug A then you may be fine. If he gives you drug B you may be fine. But if he gives you drug A and drug B together the mixture may kill you. Very little research is done into the ways drugs interact when given simultaneously.

6. Little or no research is done into the long-term effectiveness and safety of drugs which have been licensed for human use. Once a drug is on the market it can stay on the market for as long as its manufacturer is making a profit — without anyone finding out whether it really does work and is safe. Only if someone somewhere happens to notice that 75% of the patients who take that drug turn purple and explode will the drug's safety be questioned.

Since most research is paid for by drug companies (and since they have a vested interest in ensuring that none of this research is ever done) it is, I'm afraid, extremely unlikely that there will ever be any answers to these problems. None of this research would cost very much to organise.

31

Nurses have now been given legal authority to prescribe. This is lunacy and means that patients will, in future, have to take very special care to protect themselves from incompetent, prescription-happy nurses as well as incompetent, prescription-happy doctors. Nurses should dress wounds, soothe brows, make beds and provide bedpans. If they want to prescribe they should become doctors. Preferably good doctors.

The decision to allow nurses to hand out prescriptions for potentially lethal medicines was made without any extensive research being done to find out whether or not nurses could prescribe sensibly and wisely. It was done simply because there is a massive shortage of doctors, and doctors (with a six year training period) are expensive to train. No one who authorised this absurd decision seems to me to have paid enough concern to the problems that will inevitably be produced. With tens of thousands of additional prescribers, none of them as well trained as doctors (whose own training is pretty pathetic), there is no doubt that far more people will be taking far more drugs (it is not difficult to guess that the drug companies must have been behind this decision to allow nurses to prescribe), there will be far more deaths from drug side effects, far more illnesses created by drug side effects and far more dangerous drug interactions. Doctors, who receive a much lengthier training than nurses, do not prescribe drugs well. There is every reason to believe that nurses, whose training period is much shorter, will be even less competent.

32

It isn't just nurses who are going to be allowed to prescribe.

Pharmacists and other healthcare professionals are being allowed to hand out prescriptions. How long before porters and cleaners will be allowed to carry prescription pads in their overalls? (They would probably be just as competent as some doctors and most nurses.)

33

Pharmacists, whose function was for some years confined to counting out pills and has in more recent times been confined to sticking labels on packets of pills, are going to be used as second-class general practitioners; doing blood pressure checks and performing other tasks previously done by doctors. (They will do this in addition to handing out prescriptions.) The reason for this is simple: it is much cheaper and quicker to train pharmacists than it is to train doctors.

34

Don't just ignore it if you develop a rash, indigestion, tinnitus, a headache or some other possible side effect: report it to your doctor straight away. Don't stop medication without asking his advice first. Some side effects are mild and if the drug is working and helping to control or defeat a serious or life-threatening condition then the side effects may be of little consequence. But other side effects may kill. Many of the thousands who die each year could still be alive if they had taken action earlier when side effects started.

35

Organisations intended to provide information and support for patients are a wonderful idea. In the early 1970s I compiled what was, I believe, the world's first directory of such organisations. Many were small and run by determined, well-intentioned individuals who usually had a close relative suffering from the disease in question. Some of the people were best described as nutters. But they were honest nutters. Their intentions were good and the work they did was valuable. The best of these organisations helped share information and support and encouraged patients and their relatives to concentrate not on their illness but on working to reduce the impact it had on their lives.

Sadly, as with so many things in life, things have changed. And in this instance, as in so many others, they have not changed for the better.

Many organisations which exist to provide information about specific diseases are now funded by (and run on behalf of) pharmaceutical companies.

When a small organisation which used to be run from someone's spare bedroom suddenly starts offering a free phone number and providing expensively printed brochures you can bet that the brochures (and the organisation) will be promoting a product.

Does it matter that such groups are sponsored?

Well, I think it does.

The drug companies which provide sponsorship do not do so out of the goodness of their non-existent hearts; they do it for hard commercial reasons. They want to make sure that patients are told about products which are available (but which might not be suitable) and they want to be sure that warnings and problems associated with profitable products are suppressed. Eventually, there is a real risk that a group will come to depend upon the drug company's money (a sum which might not be much to the company but might be a good deal for the organisation).

If you saw that this book was sponsored by a company selling painkillers or vitamins, or that my website was sponsored by a company selling a treatment for osteoporosis you would, I hope, wonder if my words might not have been tempered in some way so as to (at the very least) not offend my sponsor. Or you might wonder which items in the book were there because the sponsor wanted them there. (It is, of course, for this reason that my books and website aren't sponsored and don't carry any advertising — welcome though such money would be. I am not worried that I might succumb to pressure to change my words. I know I wouldn't. But readers might wonder. And so the easy way to remove the suspicion is to accept no sponsorship or advertising.)

Not all organisations retain their integrity as they grow. Time and time again people start small groups and because they are inspired by my books they invite me to be patron. Then they start getting government, EU or drug company grants and my name is quickly and quietly dropped from the masthead.

36

If you take three drugs and two of them are for side effects caused by the first drug then you are probably being badly treated.

The medical profession's obsession with drugs means that many doctors still regard drug side effects as merely a reason for reaching for the prescription pad and writing out a prescription for yet another drug.

Countless millions of patients around the world are regularly given drugs which do nothing but cover up the side effects of other drugs which they are taking.

Time and time again a patient who is receiving treatment for one condition will go to a doctor complaining of new symptoms and simply be given a prescription for a new drug. Sadly, most doctors are still unaware of Coleman's 1st Law of Medicine.

It is, I believe, this basic ignorance, fostered by too strong a trust in the pharmaceutical industry, which explains why so many doctors show signs of being every bit as intelligent and percipient as living room furniture.

This problem is now so widespread that I believe that any doctor wishing to make a quick name for himself could probably obtain a staggeringly high cure rate simply by collecting patients and then encouraging them to wean themselves off their prescription medicines.

I readily acknowledge that some medicines make a valid contribution to health and that one would have to be careful when applying this unusual treatment programme but, nevertheless, I think it would work. I think one could, quite conservatively, expect a dramatic and long-term improvement in a third of the patients encouraged to stop taking their pills. I do stress, however, that stopping or cutting down pills must be done under qualified medical supervision. You might be one of those rare patients who actually needs to take prescription drugs.

37

Never, ever trust a doctor who tells you that the drug he is prescribing is free of all side effects. Leave his consulting room as quickly as you can. And never go back.

Coleman's 2nd Law Of Medicine

There is no point in having tests done unless the results will affect your treatment.

1

If your doctor wants you to have tests done ask him how the results will affect your treatment. If the results of the tests won't affect the treatment you receive (and aren't needed as a baseline against which to compare future tests) then the tests aren't worth having.

Tests and investigations are often regarded (by both doctors and patients) as being harmless. They aren't. There is no such thing as minor surgery (Coleman's 11th Law Of Medicine) and even taking blood is an operation. There are dangers inherent in every test that is performed. And there is, in addition, the danger that the result will be wrong and that your doctors will treat the test rather than treating you.

2

One of the problems with doctors doing too many tests and investigations is the fact that this overloads the laboratories where tests are done.

As I write this I have in front of me a letter from a British doctor inviting a patient to have a routine cervical smear test. 'Your result will be available from us within 12 weeks,' concludes the letter, as though this was some sort of added benefit.

Twelve weeks of worry!

What sort of feeble-spirited doctor would send out a letter like that? Don't doctors realise that patients worry about the results when they have a test done to find out whether or not they have cancer? Don't doctors realise that worrying makes people ill?

For years I have received a steady stream of letters from readers reporting that they have had to wait weeks or even months before receiving vital results after blood tests, X-rays, biopsies and other investigations. In many cases patients had to wait long periods of time to find out whether or not they had cancer. For example, it is not uncommon for tests done to find out whether women have breast cancer to take over three months to be returned to the patient's doctor. Just how this can be explained, let alone excused, I have no idea. Most test results should be obtainable within minutes or, at most, within a day or two. Any doctor who routinely expects patients to wait days, weeks or months to find out whether or not they have cancer or some other threatening disease is unthinking, barbaric and quite unfit to practise medicine. What damage does the worry do to the health of patients who need to be at their strongest? What additional damage is done to the health of worrying relatives and friends?

3

Doctors often refuse to start treatment until they have received all the test results back. If they get test results within hours or days that is fine. But in some hospitals it can take months for test results to return. If a patient with symptoms of a bladder infection provides a urine sample so that any urinary tract infection can be identified it makes sense to start the patient on treatment with an antibiotic. If the test result shows that the antibiotic prescribed was the wrong one an appropriate drug can then be prescribed. Patients sometimes die untreated because doctors will not (or dare not) try treatments until all the investigations have been completed. The threat of litigation means that doctors insist on waiting for convincing evidence before trying anything. Inevitably, this means that it is not infrequently too late to act by the time treatment is started. If, for example, there are two or three possible diagnoses available and only one of the diseases can be treated then it would seem to make sense to start the treatment for the disease which can be treated, even though laboratory evidence in support of that diagnosis might not be available. But this isn't what happens.

4

Doctors have a tendency to treat investigation results rather than patients. Don't let them do this to you. When clinical observations and laboratory findings are incompatible, the laboratory findings are wrong.

Coleman's 3rd Law Of Medicine

If the treatment doesn't work then you should consider the possibility that the diagnosis might be wrong. This is particularly true when several treatments have been tried.

1

Doctors pay far too much attention to high technology equipment these days. Probably as a result, they are often frighteningly bad at making diagnoses. A study, published in 2004, showed that major disorders are not picked up in around four out of ten patients. When doctors compared post-mortem results with the patients' medical records they discovered that out of 87 patients only 17 patients were diagnosed completely correctly. Ten of the patients might have survived if the diagnosis had been more accurate. In 15 cases major problems (such as heart attacks) were not detected.

Whoops, whoops and whoops again.

2

In 1991, one in ten hospital deaths was followed by a post mortem. In 2004 the figure had fallen to 1 in 40. When fewer post mortems are performed doctors are less likely to be embarrassed by evidence showing that they made a big mistake. Doctors are also, of course, unlikely to learn anything if they never know how wrong they were.

The number of post mortems performed has fallen for several reasons. One is undoubtedly to save expense. Another is because if there is no post mortem (and no record of the mistakes that have been made) the hospital is less likely to find itself besieged by lawyers. But the single most important reason is undoubtedly the fact that not having post mortems helps to reduce the amount of embarrassment doctors feel when their diagnoses are proved wrong.

3

Patients used to hand over their health (and their lives) to their doctors — without ever questioning what was happening to them. Today, that is a dangerous way to live. Patients who take an interest in their own health (and in the investigations and treatments that are recommended for them) may sometimes feel that the doctors and nurses who are looking after them regard them as a nuisance. But all the evidence shows clearly that such patients get better quicker, suffer fewer unpleasant side effects and live longer than patients who simply lie back passively and allow the professionals to take over.

If your doctor wants you to take a drug (and all pills, tablets, capsules, medicines, potions, creams and so on are drugs) make sure you know what to expect. If your doctor wants you to have surgery then make sure that you know what the surgery entails, what the possible consequences might be and what the alternatives are. Two really good questions to ask your doctor are: 'Would you have this treatment if you were me?' and 'Would you recommend this treatment to someone in your close family?

Learn as much as you can about any disorder from which you suffer. And learn about all the possible types of treatment available. Patients who know more about their condition than their doctors invariably do better than patients who know nothing and put all their trust in their medical advisers.

4

Common things occur commonly. It's amazing how many doctors forget this.

5

However many symptoms you've got, you (and your doctor) should always assume that there is but one cause. Only when this belief becomes impossible to sustain should you reluctantly and cautiously consider the possibility that there may be more than one thing wrong with you. And even then they are probably connected.

6

Never be afraid to ask for a second opinion. It is your life that is at stake — not a new sofa or curtains for the living room.

7

Telling your doctor that you want a second opinion will probably take a great deal of courage. Many doctors are sensitive creatures — they may show their hurt if their all-knowingness is questioned. But just remember that the stakes are high. And, if there is time, don't be afraid to check out the past record of the doctor who is going to treat you. One surgeon working in a hospital may have a survival rate which is twice as good as another surgeon working in the same hospital. If you allow the less competent surgeon to operate on you then your chances of walking out of the hospital may be halved. Those are odds you cannot and should not ignore.

8

For several months I had a persistent, nagging pain in my back. It was just about in the region of my right kidney. It didn't seem to be getting any worse but it certainly wasn't getting any better.

For a while I managed to convince myself that it was nothing more than a muscular backache caused by crouching over a keyboard. But then I noticed two additional symptoms.

I started feeling constantly 'full' — as though I had just eaten a large meal — and I found that my bladder needed emptying more often than I found entirely convenient.

When I told my general practitioner he took a routine urine sample.

And found blood.

The next step was a hospital appointment.

The ultrasound pictures showed a rather misshapen kidney. And more specialist X-ray pictures confirmed that there was something wrong. My kidney looked as though it was auditioning for a part as the hunchback of Notre Dame.

Unhappily, however, the radiologists couldn't get a really good view of my kidney. Their view was obscured by large bubbles of inconvenient gas lurking around in the coiled nooks and crannies of my intestinal loops. But they thought I had renal cancer. And I was told to prepare myself for surgery. (As an aside, when I asked a radiologist about the local surgeons I was told that one was competent but a bit rude whereas the other was pleasant but not very good.)

At my insistence I was given an appointment to go to another, larger, city hospital for even more sophisticated tests and a second opinion.

The radiologist at the large city hospital told me that there was nothing wrong with my kidney. It was, he assured me, misshapen but perfectly healthy.

I had narrowly escaped having a kidney ripped out.

But, despite all these tests, the doctors still didn't know what was wrong with me. ('You go off and enjoy yourself,' one of the doctors had said, when they still thought I had cancer. 'We'll sort this out when you get back.')

And so, after racing to the television studios to record a TV programme, and hurtling back home to write a column, I set off, as I had previously planned, to Paris.

On the plane flying over the Channel the pain in my back got much, much worse.

And I suddenly realised what was wrong.

The gas that the radiologist had spotted in my intestines had expanded because of the change in air pressure and it was the gas that was causing my pain.

And making me feel 'full' all the time.

And irritating my bowel and my bladder.

And pressing on my kidney and causing the bleeding.

There was only one explanation for this apparently bizarre set of circumstances.

I had irritable bowel syndrome.

The moment I made the diagnosis I realised just why I had acquired this most common of twenty-first century disorders.

First, I had been putting myself under an enormous amount of stress. For years I had run a series of passionate campaigns designed to spread the truth and oppose those parts of the medical establishment with which I disagreed. I had, for years, been spending twelve hours a day on my campaigns.

Second, I had changed my diet. I had cut out all meat and fish and increased the quantity of vegetables and cereals.

Irritable bowel syndrome isn't easy to control. Once you've got it then you're probably going to have symptoms for life.

But I didn't have kidney cancer.

If I hadn't had a second opinion...

Coleman's 4ᵗʰ Law Of Medicine

Screening examinations and check-ups are more profitable for doctors than for patients.

1

I have been a stern critic of screening examinations and check-ups for several decades and have, in the distant past, pointed out that well-known (and extremely profitable) forms of testing such as the cervical smear, the breast mammogram and the prostate specific antigen (psa) test for prostate cancer may, over the years, have done considerably more harm than good. Naturally, my criticisms have been met with a barrage of angry and very defensive comments from doctors who earn their living providing screening tests, and from companies which make money out of producing screening equipment. Today, the industry promoting health checks continues to promote (and profit from) them though, I am pleased to say, that a growing number of doctors now share my fear that such tests may, in the long run, do far more harm than good. For example, in 2004, a study by experts at Stanford University Medical School in the USA suggested that the psa test could not be relied upon to produce accurate results. And in recent years more and more doctors have come to accept that routine mammograms (in which the breast tissue is X-rayed) are far too dangerous and should be avoided.

It was in 1988 that I first warned about the danger of mammograms in a book called *The Health Scandal*. My criticism was, of course, greeted with howls of outrage from the medical establishment. Back then I wrote: 'There are, of course, risks in having regular X-ray examinations. No one knows yet exactly what those risks are. We will probably find out in another ten or twenty years time.'

In fact it was in 2006 that doctors finally issued a warning about mammograms, coming to precisely the conclusion I had warned about eighteen years earlier. Mammographic screening may help prevent breast cancer. But it may also cause breast cancer. Just how many women die because of the radiation they have received through mammography isn't known but it seems that the risks for younger women (women in their 30's for example) are higher than the risks for older women. (Radiation-induced cancer typically takes up to 20 years to develop so for a woman in her 80's the risks of mammography are probably somewhere between slight and negligible.) According to some estimates, out of every 10,000 women who have mammography from the age of 40 onwards between two and four will develop radiation-induced breast cancer. One of them will die as a result of this. The precise figures are unknown and depend upon the quality and amount of the radiation, the skill of the technician and other factors — probably including the general health of the woman concerned.

Does mammography cause more cancers than it helps to prevent? Would other forms of screening be safer and therefore more effective?

I don't know. This is a decision that every woman has to make for herself. I certainly don't believe that anyone knows the answers to those questions with any certainty either. Personally, if pushed for an answer, I would have to say that I believe (as I did in 1988) that mammography should be stopped until some proper long-term testing has been done. It won't be of course. The commercial and political reasons for continuing with mammography are far too powerful.

2

Mammograms have, I believe, one thing in common with vaccines. Both are examples of high technology preventive medicine introduced for profitability rather than effectiveness.

3

Men are never offered the opportunity to attend mammography screenings. And yet breast cancer does also affect men. One in every 200 patients with breast cancer is a man. How many more cases of male breast cancer would be identified if men were being screened and checked as often as women are?

4

There are three common myths about mammography:

Myth 1. Mammography reduces the incidence of breast cancer.

It doesn't. Mammography doesn't help prevent breast cancer. The very best it can do is detect breast cancer at an early stage.

Myth 2. Mammography saves lives because early detection means a better chance of surviving.

This isn't necessarily true. If there is no effective therapy then the point at which the cancer is detected will make no difference to the outcome but will merely affect the length of time that the patient knows that she has cancer. If the cancer is very slow growing and is unlikely to kill then early detection may make no difference to the outcome. For example, a type of breast cancer that is called ductal carcinoma in situ can be detected by mammography. About half the cases of this type of cancer do not seem to progress. Early detection of breast cancer (or any other type of cancer) doesn't necessarily help the patient. If the cancer will not grow, or will grow so slowly that it is no serious threat to the patient's life, early detection may do more harm than good. Treatment for the cancer (surgery or radiotherapy) may endanger the woman's life, and reduce the quality of her life, without any advantage.

Myth 3. Women who have annual mammography screening are protected from breast cancer.

Some breast cancers are very aggressive and are likely to grow extremely rapidly. These fast growing cancers are commonest in young women. An annual mammography screening, which checks the breasts just once a year, is unlikely to be of much use in detecting this type of cancer.

5

Politicians and journalists often campaign for mammography to be made available to all women. This really doesn't make any sort of sense. None of the ten randomised trials I've found suggest that mammographic screening of women in their 40's reduces breast cancer mortality. There are several reasons for this. First, women under 50 are less likely to have breast cancer than are older women. Second, when breast cancer does develop in younger women it may be fast growing (so an annual check-up may be of no use). Third, breast density is higher among young women so screening is less likely to be able to detect cancer at a curable stage.

With women who are over the age of 50 there may be some advantage in mammography, although the benefits are still questionable (especially when the risks are taken into consideration). Some studies of mammography among women over 50 have found a significant reduction in breast cancer mortality. But, on the other hand, some studies found little or no reduction in breast cancer mortality.

6

Doctors and patients are very poor at assessing risks. Both tend to worry about the wrong things. Both tend to ignore the risks associated with tests and investigations but X-ray induced cancer is a real risk that should be taken seriously.

7

Some women who have mammograms are falsely diagnosed as having breast cancer. These are known as 'false positives'. All these women will be re-investigated. Some will have surgery and will lose perfectly healthy breasts. Even biopsies can be dangerous. Apart from the psychological problems there may be wound infections, bruising, scarring and the loss of breast tissue. The risk of acquiring a serious and life-threatening antibiotic resistant infection must also be considered.

The incidence of false positives among women who have mammograms is phenomenally high. In one investigation of 26,000 women who had mammography screening for the first time, only 1 in every 10 women who tested 'positive' was subsequently found to have breast cancer. In other words out of every ten women who were diagnosed as suffering from breast cancer as a result of mammography only one actually had breast cancer. The other nine were terrified (and probably scarred) entirely unnecessarily. Among younger women the incidence of false positives is even higher. Every year in America around 300,000 women with perfectly healthy breasts have unnecessary biopsies. It has been suggested that women whose breasts are physically damaged may be more likely to develop cancer. How many of those 300,000 will develop breast cancer as a result of their biopsies? How many will die of infection?

8

Many women who, as a result of mammography, are diagnosed as suffering from breast cancer, and who subsequently have surgery and radiotherapy, believe that their lives have been saved by their surgeons and oncologists. These women often become earnest advocates of mammography.

However, the sad truth is that many of these women have gained nothing from surgery and radiotherapy but have, on the contrary, lost a good deal as a result of their experience.

Mammography enables doctors to pick up ductal carcinoma in situ, a type of breast cancer which would have probably never been noticed in the woman's lifetime except for the mammogram.

This type of cancer is confined to the milk ducts within the breast and has not spread to surrounding tissue. It cannot be detected by a breast examination (even one performed by a skilled and experienced doctor) but will be picked up on a mammogram.

Most breast cancers detected by mammography among women in their 30's, and around 40% of breast cancers detected by mammography among women in their 40s, are ductal carcinomas in situ.

There are still gaps in our knowledge about ductal carcinoma in situ but many doctors believe that more often than not this type of cancer never spreads. In these instances, mammography helps doctors pick up, and treat, an entirely harmless abnormality. In some women (and the figures aren't defined) ductal carcinoma in situ does eventually spread and become invasive cancer. This may, however, take 20 to 30 years.

9

Women who are diagnosed with breast cancer when they don't have it at all (false positives) and women who have breast cancer which is no threat to their lives (probably most of the women with ductal carcinoma in situ) pay a high price for undergoing mammography screening. For these women the unnecessary treatment they receive, and the anxiety they must suffer, may decrease both the quality and extent of their lives.

Here then, is more evidence that mammography can kill as well as save lives.

10

There is another group of women who suffer as a result of mammography.

These are the women (known as false negatives) who are wrongly assured that they do not have breast cancer.

The false negative rate for mammography is between 5% and 20% with the higher figure relating to younger women.

So, out of 100 women who have breast cancer and have mammography screening, up to 20 will be wrongly told that they are perfectly healthy and need not worry. How many of these relieved and falsely reassured women will then ignore the lumps they may subsequently feel in their breasts? How many will die because they have been falsely reassured?

I have no idea.

Nor, I suspect, has anyone else.

11

Women are entitled to have access to all the facts before making a decision about whether or not to undergo mammography. I wonder how many are told of all the hazards. Sadly, the evidence I have seen suggests that most of the doctors and charities and commercial screening groups who promote and make money out of mammography don't tell women of these risks, complications and uncertainties.

Doctors and organisations who make money out of providing mammography have a vested interest in getting as many women as they can to take part in mammography. One recent survey reported that 92% of women said they believed that mammography cannot harm women who don't have breast cancer. None of the women surveyed seemed aware of all the hazards I have outlined here. Neither leaflets published by organisations offering mammography, nor journalists offering allegedly independent comments on mammography, discuss the risks.

12

'When trouble is sensed well in advance it can easily be remedied: if you wait for it to show itself any medicine will be too late because the disease will have become incurable. As the doctors say of a wasting disease, to start with it is easy to cure but difficult to diagnose; after a time, unless it has been diagnosed and treated at the outset, it becomes easy to diagnose but difficult to cure.'

Niccolo Machiavelli

Coleman's 5th Law Of Medicine

It is doctors, not patients, who need annual check-ups.

1

Along with cancer and circulatory disease, doctors are now one of the three most important causes of death and injury. Incompetent or careless doctors cause a horrifying amount of death or injury.

In America the Public Citizen Health Research Group has shown that 'more than 100,000 people are killed or injured a year by negligent medical care'. The real figure is probably considerably higher than this and there can be little doubt that many of the injuries and deaths among patients are caused by simple, straightforward incompetence rather than bad luck or unforeseen complications.

When doctors from the Harvard School of Public Health studied what happened to more than 30,000 patents admitted to acute care hospitals in New York they found that nearly 4% of them suffered unintended injuries in the course of their treatment and that 14% of the patients died of their injuries. This survey concluded that nearly 200,000 people die each year in America as a result of medical accidents. It is clear, therefore, that doctors kill vastly more innocent people than terrorists do. What sort of panic would political leaders be in if terrorists regularly killed 200,000 Americans every year?

2

Carotid endarterectomies — in which deposits are removed from the arteries in the neck — are currently fashionable in America where doctors earn $1.5 billion a year performing them. But when a study of carotid endarterectomies was recently completed it was found that 64% of these operations were either unjustified or of debatable value because the symptoms were not severe enough to justify the risks of the operation.

For pacemaker implants the equivalent figure is 56%.

Coronary bypass operations are immensely popular among heart surgeons (and extremely profitable) but a major study conducted in Europe showed that many patients who don't have surgery live longer than those who do. In 1990 American surgeons performed 350,000 coronary bypass operations and charged $14 billion for them. When one researcher studied 300 patients who had had bypass operations at several hospitals in California he discovered that 14% of the patients would have thrived as well without surgery as with it while another 30% were borderline.

Around 50% of lower back disc operations and up to 70% of hysterectomies are probably unnecessary. In America the death toll from unnecessary surgery alone has been estimated to be as high as 80,000 patients per year. (That's on top of the figure of 200,000 I reported above.)

3

Two Irish doctors reported in the *British Medical Journal* that 20% of British patients who have slightly raised blood pressure are treated unnecessarily with drugs. A British Royal College of Radiologists Working Party reported that at least a fifth of radiological examinations carried out in National Health Service hospitals were clinically unhelpful. In Britain the Institute of Economic Affairs claimed that inexperienced doctors in casualty units kill at least one thousand patients a year.

4

Doctors (egged on by drug companies) often claim that it is thanks to them that we are all living longer these days. There are two errors in this apparently simple claim. The first is that there is absolutely no evidence to show that we are all living longer (indeed the evidence suggests the opposite). The second error lies in the claim that drug companies and doctors have improved our general health. That's baloney too.

5

The evidence shows that there really hasn't been much change in life expectation in recent years. (After all, way back in biblical times, ordinary folk were encouraged to expect a life-span of three score and ten.)

Drug companies and doctors like to take all the credit for the alleged improvement in our life expectation (it helps to excuse their foibles and excesses) but the truth is that our longevity is a myth.

The truth is that cleaner drinking water, and better sewage facilities (introduced in the 19th century) resulted in a fall in infant mortality levels.

6

Imagine a family of five. If four members of the family live to be 70 but the fifth dies as an infant then the average life expectancy (ignoring the age at which the infant dies) will be 56. But if all five live to the age of 65 the average life expectancy will be 65.

Reducing infant mortality has made a tremendous difference to overall life expectancy figures.

7

It is sometimes argued that the fact that there are more old people around these days proves that people are living longer. This is, of course, utter nonsense. The proportion of older people in our communities has increased because couples are having fewer children.

This is partly because the fall in infant mortality means that it is no longer necessary to have twelve children as a hedge against early deaths, partly because of the ready availability of effective contraception and partly because high taxes mean that most young working couples cannot afford many children.

8

Look into any nursing home during the last few decades and you will have seen a tremendous preponderance of women. Historically, this is a fairly new phenomenon.

In my book *How To Live Longer* I pointed out that there is no reason at all why women should live longer than men. There are no anatomical or physiological reasons for the huge difference which exists in life expectation between the two sexes. In *How To Live Longer* I explained my theory that women in the 20th century were living longer for several main reasons:

1. Up until a few decades ago most women didn't smoke.

2. Up until a few decades ago most women didn't go out to work (and have to cope with all the associated physical and mental stresses).

3. Up until a few decades ago most women were allowed to regard themselves as the 'gentle' or 'weaker' sex. Significant worries about the household were the province of the man of the house.

4. Up until a few decades ago most women had jobs (such as looking after the home) which involved regular exercise. Walking to the shops and running up and down stairs might not be fun but it is exercise. Men, on the other hand, were involved in jobs which tended to mar their health. Men with manual work were exposed to asbestos or coal dust. Men with sedentary jobs put on excess weight and developed circulatory disease.

These are generalisations, of course. But, like all generalisations, they are broadly accurate.

In *How To Live Longer* I forecast that the difference in life expectation between men and women would, for fairly obvious reasons, start to fall.

And it's already happening.

The difference in life expectation between men and women is narrowing quite rapidly. By the middle of the 21st century life expectation for the two sexes will be much the same.

But it won't be male life expectation which has improved.

It will be female life expectation which will have fallen.

The few doctors who have noticed this change seem to have been surprised by it.

No effort has been put into explaining to women why they are not living as long as their mothers.

9

A big chunk of doctors are crooks who would prescribe arsenic if they got a free pen from a drug company making arsenic tablets. Many more don't know (and wouldn't dare guess) what day of the week it is unless a drug company representative told them.

10

Some people insist that their doctor is very good.

They probably mean that he is kind and courteous.

How do they know, really, really know, whether or not their doctor is truly competent?

It's very difficult to assess the knowledge and wisdom of a doctor.

Especially, if he smiles, is polite and seems to care.

11

Doctors are now a major cause of illness and death. Study the statistics and it becomes clear that throughout the 'civilised' world doctors are right up there alongside heart disease and cancer as the big-time killers of the twenty-first century.

A study in Australia showed that 470,000 Australian men, women and children are admitted to hospital every year because they have been made ill by doctors. The figures also show that every year 280,000 patients who are admitted to hospital suffer a temporary disability as a result of their health care. Around 50,000 of these suffer permanent disabilities. A staggering 18,000 Australians die annually as a result of medical errors, drug toxicity, surgical errors and general medical mismanagement. What a terrible indictment of the medical profession.

Figures in Europe are no better. In my book *Betrayal of Trust* I explained why one in six British hospital patients is in hospital and receiving treatment because he or she has been made ill by doctors.

The story is the same the whole world over and doctors no longer seem to deny any of this. No one in the medical profession has ever disputed my research or this figure. Indeed, when I did a radio broadcast to talk about my book the producers of the programme invited a representative of the British Medical Association into the studio. When I made the point that one in six patients in hospital is there because doctors have created an illness, this doctor's response to my attack on the profession we share was unforgettable. 'The positive thought we can take from this,' he said in his best bedside manner, 'is that five out of every six patients in hospital are *not* there because they have been made ill by doctors.'

(No, I could hardly believe it either. But I listened to a tape of the programme afterwards and that is exactly what he said.)

12

Around half of all the 'adverse effects' associated with doctors are clearly and readily preventable and are usually a result of ignorance or incompetence or a mixture of both. The rest would be preventable with a little care and thought (and some better research).

13

Today's doctors may laugh at the surgeons who chopped out lengths of bowel to treat constipation or who cut out pieces of brain to treat hysteria, but to future generations many current practices will seem no easier to understand. Around the world there are still hundreds of doctors chopping out lengths of bowel, putting staples in stomachs or wiring up jaws to treat patients who eat too much. There are still hundreds of doctors giving patients electric shocks because they are depressed or chopping out bits and pieces of brain to treat problems as varied as schizophrenia, anxiety and drug addiction. Most alarming of all, perhaps, is the fact that as hospitals are filled with increasingly sophisticated equipment (which doctors and technicians often do not entirely understand) so the opportunities for error are constantly being enhanced. For example, there have been several reports showing that patients receiving radiation treatment have been given the wrong dosage.

14

Surveys of junior hospital doctors regularly show an alarming ignorance about drugs, prescription writing and the performance of simple, practical procedures. The basic problem is that medical schools are run by people who are academics rather than practical physicians. Medical schools should sack all their earnest, super-specialists (who have never seen a case of measles or stood in a patient's bedroom) and hire retired family doctors as teachers.

15

It was estimated in one medical publication that three quarters of surgeons were still using hernia repair techniques which were regarded internationally as obsolete.

Once a surgeon has got a job he is likely to stay set in his ways. Over the years the only thing that will change is that he will acquire an increasing number of prejudices and bad habits.

16

The overuse of medical facilities — particularly surgery — is a common cause of unnecessary injury and death. When a patient is likely to die if an operation is not performed the risks associated with the operation may be acceptable. But when procedures are performed unnecessarily the risks become unacceptable.

According to *Fortune* magazine American hospitals now try to attract doctors who will bring in patients likely to run up substantial bills. Centres offering investigative facilities often offer lucrative partnerships to doctors who are prepared to promise to make lots of referrals.

Research in British hospitals has shown that pregnant women who are in private beds in NHS hospitals are twice as likely to have their babies by Caesarian section as women in NHS beds. Could this possibly be due to the fact that surgeons looking after private patients can charge a hefty extra fee for delivering a baby by Caesarian section? If not, what other explanation can you think of?

17

Doctors, nurses, drug companies and hospitals are now one of the three or four main causes of death and serious illness in all the so-called 'developed' countries. As a cause of death and serious illness, iatrogenic diseases (disorders caused by doctors and hospitals) are up there alongside cancer and circulatory disorders (such as strokes and heart attacks).

The medical profession in general, and the medical establishment in particular, turns a blind eye and does nothing about the problems which they know exist.

The quality of care in hospitals is falling as a result of overprescribing, an over-emphasis on political correctness, new employment law (which makes it virtually impossible to sack an incompetent nurse or doctor), over bureaucratisation, a failure to understand the importance of simple hygiene, endless varieties of intrusive and unhelpful legislation and a wild, unbridled enthusiasm for high technology.

There is a grave tendency among doctors (as among all other apparently intelligent members of our society) to use computers whenever possible. This is, of course, a sign of rank stupidity. Computers should only be used when they will help you do something better — not because they can do something. Doctors tend to use computers to do things that computers *can* do, rather than to use them to do things they *want* them to do. This is a result of the fact that so-called 'information technology' people are, generally, keen for doctors (and everyone else) to use their computers to do whatever it is they have made them able to do and not to redesign computers to do what people want them to do. (No one could accuse me of being a technophobe. I bought my first computer in the 80's and had my first website presence at the same time. I have been using a mobile telephone since the mid 1980s and a fax machine just as long. I've used a palm-sized computer for over a decade.) But the wild enthusiasm for, and over-reliance on, anything which has a plug on the end of it has created massive problems and, I have no doubt, has resulted in more deaths than it has saved lives.

In practice, computers are merely typewriters which go wrong a lot and the Internet, a tool for governments rather than individuals, has proved most successful as a replacement for classified advertising sections of local newspapers and as a source of pornographic material. One of the biggest problems with the Internet is that medical students and young doctors are learning to rely for research on computerised search engines. This is very dangerous since when you research a subject on a computer's search engine there is a real danger that you will be fed material which has gained its position on the list because a drug company has paid for it to be there or because some computer nerd has manipulated its position on the list. Many young doctors don't realise that search engines are 'bent' and unreliable. Search engines pose one of the greatest of all the threats to what remains of the medical profession's badly damaged independence and indeed, to the safety and security of patients everywhere. Doctors (and others) who rely on search engines to do their research are doomed to receive information which is at best doubtful and at worst downright corrupt.

18

The regulators who are supposed to protect patients from dishonest or disreputable doctors seem generally unconcerned with things which really should concern them. When newspapers reported that a large drug company had been reprimanded by the industry's own 'watchdog' for paying doctors to switch patients from rival medicines to its own product I saw no suggestion that the doctors involved might be subjected to professional discipline. These, remember, were doctors who had accepted bribes to change their patients' medication.

Politicians do nothing lest they upset the pharmaceutical companies (which bluff by threatening to move their operations to other countries if anything is done to damage their profits).

And hospital administrators do nothing because they don't know — and possibly don't want to know — the truth. Administrators have soaked up all the power but they have refused to accept any of the responsibility.

19

Most people recognise the damage that other doctors can do but like to think that their doctor is an honourable exception. This is entirely understandable. After all, we all like to think that our relationship with our own doctor is special and that we have chosen someone reliable and knowledgeable to look after us.

We like to think of our doctor as a personal and family friend. We all need to put some trust in the health care professionals upon whom we rely when we are ill.

But it is just as dangerous to assume that your doctor is entirely safe, sensible, knowledgeable, competent and error free as it would be to assume that you do not need to take care when driving, on the spurious grounds that road accidents only ever affect other people.

20

Most doctors would rather admit to having made a mistake than give credit to a non-orthodox treatment. Cures resulting from alternative treatments are sometimes dismissed as 'miracles' or dismissed as spontaneous remissions. More commonly doctors will claim that it was their treatment (however long ago it was given) which was responsible for the improvement. The cure of a patient by a new and alternative (or complementary) remedy will be credited to the patient's previous medical attendants. Of course, when a patient dies after trying a new and alternative remedy the failure will be blamed entirely on the alternative therapy.

This is a variation on an old saying which runs something like this: 'When nature cures the doctor takes the credit; when nature fails, nature takes the blame.'

21

Given a choice between an old and experienced doctor who is out of touch with modern developments, and a young doctor who is fresh out of medical school and who knows all the latest jargon, the patient who puts experience ahead of knowledge will benefit.

22

Doctors are now part of the establishment and tend, therefore, to oppose genuine innovation and original thought. Anyone offering a new and genuinely constructive insight into a healthcare problem is likely to be attacked, reviled and discredited. This is stupid and indefensible. But it is the way it is.

23

Any doctor who tells you that you will need to take pills for life is an unimaginative (and probably ill-informed) buffoon.

24

Most medical treatments are untried and have never been proved to be any good at all. Even drug treatments which are well-established have still not yet been properly thought out or evaluated. Prejudice and superstition are hardly a sound basis for good science.

25

Drugs are wildly over-prescribed, both by hospital doctors and by general practitioners. It is now over 30 years since I first exposed the dangers of benzodiazepines and 15 years since a British Government admitted that it had introduced new legislation as a result of my campaign to expose the dangers of these drugs. (A campaign which was vociferously opposed by the medical establishment.) But benzodiazepines are still over-prescribed and they are still prescribed badly, without thought and without awareness of the often disastrous consequences for patients. Vast numbers of other drugs, including antibiotics and painkillers as well as anti-depressants, are frequently over-prescribed. Vaccines are also a major cause of illness and death.

26

As I proved in my evidence to a House of Lords select committee, animal experiments are done not to help patients but to improve drug company profits. The drug industry's reliance on animal experiments has led to the deaths of countless thousands of patients.

27

Doctors and hospitals are often appallingly and inexcusably slow. Delays usually do nothing to damage hospital success rates. A patient is only officially recorded as suffering from cancer on the date when he or she is officially diagnosed.

28

Doctors save lives but they also kill people.

There is nothing new in that.

Doctors have always made mistakes and there have always been patients who have died as a result of medical ignorance or incompetence.

But we have now reached the point where, on balance, many well-meaning doctors in general practice and many highly-trained, well-equipped specialists working in hospitals do more harm than good. Through a mixture of ignorance and incompetence doctors are killing more people than they are saving and they are causing more illness and more discomfort than they are alleviating.

It is true, of course, that doctors save thousands of lives by prescribing life-saving drugs such as antibiotics and by performing essential life-saving surgery on road accident victims.

But the tragedy is that the good which doctors do is often far outweighed by the bad. What is even more worrying is the fact that the epidemic of iatrogenic disease (disease caused by doctors) which has scarred medical practice for decades has been steadily getting worse. Today most of us would, most of the time, be better off without a medical profession.

29

A former Director General of the World Health Organisation startled the medical establishment by stating that: 'the major and most expensive part of medical knowledge as applied today appears to be more for the satisfaction of the health professions than for the benefit of the consumers of health care'. The evidence certainly supports that apparently controversial view.

Consider, for example, what happens when doctors go on strike and leave patients to cope without professional medical help. You might imagine that people would be dying like flies in autumn. Not a bit of it. When doctors in Israel went on strike for a month admissions to hospital dropped by eighty five per cent, with only the most urgent cases being admitted, but despite this the death rate in Israel dropped by fifty per cent — the largest drop since the previous doctors' strike twenty years earlier — to its lowest ever recorded level. Much the same thing has happened wherever doctors have gone on strike. In Bogota, Colombia doctors went on strike for fifty two days and there was a thirty five per cent fall in the mortality rate. In Los Angeles a doctors' strike resulted in an eighteen per cent reduction in the death rate. During the strike there were sixty per cent fewer operations in seventeen major hospitals. After the strike was over the death rate went back up to normal.

Whatever statistics are consulted the conclusion has to be the same. Doctors are a hazard rather than an asset to any community.

In Britain the death rate of working men over fifty years of age was higher in the 1970s than it was in the 1930s. The British were never healthier than they were during the Second World War.

Figures published by the United States Bureau of Census show that thirty three per cent of the people born in 1907 could expect to live to the age of seventy five whereas thirty three per cent of the people born in 1977 could expect to live to the age of eighty. Remove the improvements produced by better living conditions and fewer deaths during or just after childbirth and it becomes clear that doctors, drug companies and hospitals cannot possibly have had any useful effect on life expectancy. Indeed, the figures show that there has been an increase in mortality rates among the middle aged and an increase in the incidence of disabling disorders such as diabetes and arthritis.

Could there be some other explanation for this dispiriting phenomenon? Hardly. When you look at the quality of medical care it becomes clear that it must be doctors who are responsible for the decline in health.

30

So far I have written only about general practitioners. But it isn't only family doctors who need to be better trained. A report published in the *Journal of the Royal Society of Medicine* concluded that many hospital patients who suffer heart attacks die during the 'confused and disorganised charades' of attempts to save them because hospital doctors do not know how to give emergency resuscitation.

Even more worrying was an editorial published in the *British Medical Journal* which stated that: 'only one per cent of the articles in medical journals are scientifically sound' and that 'only about fifteen per cent of medical interventions are supported by solid scientific evidence'. In other words the majority of treatments are completely untried and when a doctor writes out a prescription or sticks a knife into a patient neither he nor anyone else has much of an idea about what will happen next.

31

There are many reasons why doctors are currently doing so much harm to their patients but among them is undoubtedly the fact that while doctors are now in possession of technologies and techniques which are powerful the profession's relationship with patients is still based on the theory that in order to do good the average doctor must rely on the fear and respect of his patients.

When doctors didn't have powerful drugs to hand out they relied heavily upon the mystique of being a 'doctor'. The mysticism and the witchcraft long associated with the practice of medicine were important parts of the healing process. Because he knew that the pills and potions he prescribed had very little intrinsic value, a doctor had to convince his patients that he knew what he was doing and that he had faith that the remedies he was using would work. The doctor knew that if his patients believed that they were going to get better then many of them would — even if they were only given some primitive and entirely useless concoction. The power of the placebo is well documented — and even quite severe pains can be controlled with sugar pills if the doctor giving out the sugar pills is convincing.

Giving the patient a prescription was an important ritual; it was offering the patient a part of the doctor to take with him and the important thing was to get the patient to believe that it would do him some good. The old-fashioned witch doctors were fearful. So were

Victorian physicians and surgeons. Patients accepted what their doctors told them as though it was gospel.

But today doctors have powerful and potentially lethal drugs and treatments at their disposal and the old-fashioned mystique is dangerous.

Patients can be too easily tempted to ask for or expect drugs and doctors can far too easily trick themselves into thinking that a prescription is necessary. When drugs were ineffective and harmless it didn't matter if doctors gave out drugs to every patient they saw. (Indeed the apothecaries — the original general practitioners — had to give drugs to all their patients since they earned their living through dispensing and were not allowed to charge fees simply for providing advice). But today although drugs are so powerful that they should be used cautiously and only when absolutely essential, old habits still persist and four out of five consultations in general practice end with the doctor handing over a prescription (although far fewer patients expect to get a prescription and most would almost certainly be happier if they left the surgery without one). The result is that we have become a nation of pill swallowers. At any one time six out of ten people in most Westernised countries will be taking a drug of some kind. It is hardly surprising that there has been an explosion in iatrogenic disease.

There is no easy, slick solution to this massive problem.

But there are some things we can do to restore some sense to health care and to reduce the appalling incidence of iatrogenic disease.

First, we need to humanise doctors — by stripping away some of their power and authority. Normally assertive and strong individuals who would confront or argue with almost anyone else they might come into contact with often find it difficult to argue with or to confront or question doctors because they have always been encouraged to regard members of the medical profession as 'different'. Doctors are treated with reverence rather than simple respect and that is a terribly unhealthy state of affairs. In the interests of good health doctors should throw away all the symbols of authority they currently use — such as the white coat.

And patients must start treating doctors more critically; they must be more demanding, more questioning and more assertive. The evidence shows that assertive patients live longer are less likely to be killed by incompetence. Patients need to be encouraged to take back responsibility for their own health and to learn to regard doctors as technicians — to be consulted but to be regarded with the variety of scepticism currently reserved for garage mechanics.

Third, and perhaps most important of all, we need also to make a genuine effort to separate the medical profession from the drugs industry. During the last few decades the two have become far too closely intertwined and today the drug industry dominates the profession; members of the medical establishment are far too uncritical of the industry. As I wrote in my first book *The Medicine Men* back in 1975 it is difficult to see how a group of people who get all their information and instructions from an industry can call themselves a profession. The little that doctors do learn about new treatments usually comes from the companies promoting their products. We need to encourage doctors to take a more cynical and sceptical look at the claims made by the big drug companies.

32

People who take drugs (and the doctors who prescribe them) still don't recognise that any symptoms which
. develop after a drug is given are probably caused by the drug.

Denying or ignoring the link between drugs and side effects is like being hit on the head by a brick and failing to recognise the link between the brick and the headache.

33

Governments need to introduce annual tests for doctors. We don't allow old cars onto the roads unless they pass a safety test. Airline pilots have to undergo regular tests. We should not allow old surgeons into the operating theatre unless they have shown that they have made some effort to keep up-to-date. Old physicians whose knowledge has passed its sell-by-date should be forcibly retired.

Doctors have a tremendous position of power and can probably do more harm than any other group of individuals in the community. But once a man or woman receives a degree certificate he or she is given a licence for life. Who would willingly fly in a plane piloted by a man who had passed his exam 50 years earlier and had not made any attempt to keep up-to-date? How many people would be happy to fly in Concorde with a pilot who was trained in a Tiger Moth — and had never had a course to update his knowledge?

Doctors should be examined annually to make sure that they keep up-to-date.

The analogy is an accurate one.

Thousands of today's doctors were trained and qualified long before most of the available modern drugs were put on the market. They neither know about nor understand the drugs they prescribe. It is this lack of independent knowledge which so often explains bizarre prescribing practices. There are an estimated 30,000 drugs available in the world. It is impossible for the average doctor to have a working knowledge of more than around 50 of those. Doctors who prescribe brand new drugs without studying the contraindications, possible side effects and interactions are putting their patients at risk.

34

All doctors should be taught to ask themselves a series of very basic questions.

1. Is the possible advantage to this patient of this treatment worth the associated risk?
One in six patients in hospital is there because he or she has been injured by a doctor. When a patient is injured by a treatment that may have saved his life then the risk is worth taking. But when a patient is injured by an unnecessary treatment the risk is not acceptable. Doctors must be taught about the risks associated with modern forms of treatment.

2. Should I interfere or do nothing?
Doing nothing is sometimes the bravest option of all. It takes a good doctor to have faith in the body's own healing powers. Many doctors like to interfere so that they can take the credit when the patient gets better.

3. What are the main priorities and main risks here?
Sorting out priorities is vital. Relieving pain is sometimes forgotten by doctors — though, to patients, relieving pain is often a number one priority.

4. What would I do (or what would I want done) if the patient was someone I loved? How would I like to be treated?

These are key questions all doctors should ask themselves every time they see a patient. Sadly, they are, I suspect, questions which are often forgotten.

35

In the summer of 2006, plans were announced in Britain for doctors to be relicensed every five years against standards drawn up by various parts of the establishment. Doctors would be assessed by a network of specially appointed affiliates who would be involved in the revalidation of doctors and who would work in harness with professional regulators.

Oh dear.

Such a scheme is destined to ensure that the worst doctors remain in practice while imaginative, caring doctors find themselves removed from the medical register.

The system will fail patients because it is within the medical establishment that the faults lie.

The best way to measure the effectiveness of doctors is to compare their success rates.

A good doctor is a doctor whose patients live long, healthy lives. A bad doctor is a doctor whose patients live short, unhealthy lives.

It should not be impossible to find a simple way to measure and compare the effectiveness of doctors in keeping their patients healthy and alive.

36

Some doctors aren't simply in need of light intellectual maintenance. Some manage to practise without any qualifications at all. Fake doctors are commoner than you might imagine.

In America a hoax psychiatrist persuaded 10 married women to have sex with total strangers.

He telephoned a hundred women at random and claimed to be a psychiatrist secretly treating their husbands for sexual problems. He told them that they should leave the house and come back with the first man they could find and await further instructions. In a second call he told the women — and the strangers they'd brought home — to have sex. He claimed it would help cure the husband's problem.

Ninety women who'd been telephoned refused to follow the hoaxer's instructions. But ten did as they were told.

In Italy a hospital found that one of its top brain surgeons wasn't even qualified as a doctor.

In England a meat salesman performed 14 operations in just 24 days while a biology teacher posed as a gynaecologist for 6 months before getting caught.

How long do you think you'd last? How convincing would you be as a doctor? Try this quiz for fun:

There is one correct answer to each of the following questions... choose the one you think is right and then check your score.

1. What would you prescribe kaolin for?
   a) a headache
   b) a tummy upset
   c) an ear infection

2. One of these drugs is an antibiotic — but which?
   a) thiamine
   b) tetracycline
   c) theophylline

3. What would you use to listen to a patient's chest?
   a) sphygmomanometer
   b) ophthalmoscope
   c) stethoscope

4. Which of these hospital specialists deals with skin problems?
   a) gynaecologist
   b) dermatologist
   c) radiologist

5. How many moles are there on the average human body?
   a) 20
   b) 2
   c) 200

6. What is the correct spelling?
   a) diarhoea
   b) diarrhoea
   c) diarrhoea

7. Which of these drugs would you prescribe for someone in pain?
   a) morphine
   b) penicillin
   c) caffeine

8. The tubes which connect your kidneys to your bladder are called
   a) catheters
   b) urethras
   c) ureters

9. If you look at a bright light your pupils will
   a) atrophy
   b) constrict
   c) dilate

10. Where is the thickest skin on your body?
   a) on your eyelids
   b) on the soles of your feet
   c) on your bottom

11. What is the name of the substance that changes the colour of your skin when you get a suntan?
   a) lymph
   b) noradrenalin
   c) melanin

12. The average human heart is roughly the size of:
   a) a table tennis ball
   b) a tennis ball
   c) a football

13. What is the name of the gland that produces the hormone insulin?
   a) the duodenum
   b) the pituitary
   c) the pancreas

14. How much blood does your body contain?
   a) 10 pints
   b) 20 pints
   c) 30 pints

The correct answers are:
1 b, 2 b, 3 c, 4 b, 5 a, 6 b, 7 a, 8 c, 9 b, 10 b, 11 c, 12 b, 13 c, 14 a.

* If you got 12 or more right — order your brass plate now!
* If you got 8 to 11 right — dodgy, you wouldn't last a week
* If you got 7 or less right — no chance, with a little practice maybe you could masquerade as a bedpan washer

37

If it isn't an emergency, always take time to study all the options. (And that includes the use of alternative or complementary medicine.)

38

In order to understand exactly why doctors are doing so much harm it is first of all necessary to demolish a very basic medical myth: that medicine is a science. Most doctors aren't scientists, most scientists aren't doctors and medicine is (still) a very unscientific discipline.

Doctors, medical researchers and drug companies like to persuade all present and potential consumers of health care that medicine is a science which has advanced beyond the mystical incantations and witch doctor remedies of the past.

But modern medicine is not a science and modern clinicians and medical researchers are not scientists.

39

The best remedy is often to do nothing but wait, watch carefully and see what happens before intervening. Doctors do not feel comfortable with this; they are trained to intervene quickly and frequently. How can a doctor claim the credit (or a fee) if he hasn't done something?

40

Doctors have begun to understand and accept the influence the mind has over the body. But few have, as yet, any idea of the importance of the spirit. No one in the health care business is likely to provide you with the spiritual guidance you need to find your way through the maze of modern life; through the conflicts and contradictions, frustrations and injustices which are now a part of our existence and which are, to a very large extent, responsible for much of the illness from which we suffer, and (for example) for the fact that the incidence of suicide has, for decades, been increasing dramatically.

41

Drug companies and politicians spend a fortune on research to find new drugs. Drug companies do this because it's how they make money. Doctors encourage them to do it because they are heavily bribed to support the drug industry in anything it does. And politicians support it (and spend public money on it) because they'll support anything if the campaign contributions (and tax bills) are big enough. Of course, one way or another the final bill for all this research will end up on our mat.

But the truth is that most of the research done by and for drug companies is a waste of time and money. It's such a misdirection of resources that it's pretty much like a race car team spending 99% of its budget on wing mirror technology.

Medical researchers, for example, tend to ignore that the power of your mind can have a dramatic effect on your health. (I dealt with this in detail in my book *Mindpower*). Your mind can make you ill and it can keep you well. It can also help make you well when you fall ill. It is, to a large extent, your state of mind which determines how successfully you cope with the stress in your life — and how well you will recover from illness.

There is another often overlooked and invariably forgotten truth about staying healthy without drugs. And that involves the power of love.

Your relationships with the people around you — and, in particular, with the people who are close to you — are vital for your health. If there isn't enough emotional love, physical love and spiritual love in your life your health will suffer.

Doctors are missing the point when they concentrate all their efforts on repairing the malfunctioning human organism. What they should spend at least some of their time on (but don't) is teaching us the importance of building and maintaining loving relationships. Few things have such a great impact on the quality (and length) of our lives as the amount of love we give and receive.

We are frequently told about the significance of genetic influences. If you have a family history of heart disease then you'll probably be warned by your doctor that you are very much at risk of developing heart disease.

That is perfectly true.

But, in general terms, the influence of genetics (in other words family history) on our lives is small when compared to the extent to which our health and longevity is influenced by the amount of love we experience. Love and intimacy are pretty well impossible to measure in scientific terms and that means that doctors ignore them. But that doesn't mean that those factors aren't important.

I first realised just how important intimacy and love can be when I was a young general practitioner back in the early 1970s. Two of my earliest patients were an elderly couple who had survived a German concentration camp together. They were frail and weak but as close as any couple can possibly be. They did absolutely everything together. Their lives were totally intertwined. And then one day he had a heart attack and died. He had suffered with a malfunctioning heart for years so, in a way, it wasn't much of a surprise. Five days later she died. That was a surprise. I can't remember what I put on the death certificate but it seemed to me that she died of a broken heart. I have no doubt whatsoever that she died simply and solely because her reason for living had gone.

That was the first time I came across the real physical significance of love and intimacy. I realised that this couple's love for one another kept them both alive through great hardships — and for much longer than they would have lived had they been alone. After a little research I discovered that this sort of thing happens quite often. When one half of a loving couple dies the other half will often follow quite quickly — even though there may be no obvious illness.

Sadly, very few doctors will admit that the amount of love and intimacy in your life can have an impact on your health. Few doctors seem to realise just how damaging loneliness can be — and just how common it is. Faced with a patient with heart disease the vast majority of doctors would simply reach for their prescription pad. Few, if any, would give their patient advice about changing their diet and building up better and stronger relationships. And yet there is clear evidence showing that the patient who changes his lifestyle can cure his heart disease and heal himself. Plus there are no side effects. Drug therapy tends only to treat the symptoms — it doesn't cure and it certainly doesn't heal. And the side effects of drug therapy can be catastrophic. But doctors reach for their prescription pads because that is what they have been taught to do — and it's what the drug industry wants them to do.

Doctors, who usually only know what the drug companies tell them, probably don't know that there is more rock solid scientific evidence showing the influence of love and food on health than there is showing the value of many of the drugs they so willingly prescribe.

Here is a brief summary of just some of the evidence which shows that love and intimacy can, and do, have a dramatic influence on our health.

1. Researchers at Yale University studied 159 patients and showed that men and women who felt the most loved had much less blockage in the arteries of their hearts. The researchers found that patients who felt loved were healthier than patients who didn't.

2. In Sweden researchers who studied 131 women showed that women who had deep emotional relationships had less coronary artery blockage than women who didn't.

3. American researchers who studied nearly 10,000 married men showed that men who answered 'yes' to the question 'Does Your Wife Show You Her Love?' had significantly less angina (heart pain) than men who did not have a loving wife — even if they might be thought to be more at risk of developing heart disease because of their ages, blood cholesterol levels, blood pressure readings and so on. 'The wife's love and support ...apparently reduces the risk of angina pectoris even if the presence of high risk factors,' concluded the researchers.

4. A study of 8,500 men showed that those who had loving wives had half the risk of developing duodenal ulcers as the men who did not have loving wives. Men who admitted that they did not think their wives loved them had three times as many ulcers as men who said their wives showed them love and support.

A surprising number of other research programmes have come to the same conclusions. And the message here is clear.

If you have a loving relationship with another human being (or, failing that, an animal) then you are far more likely to stay healthy than if you don't.

It is also clear that it is vitally important that you tell the people you love just how you feel about them. Say the words 'I love you' (and mean them) and you are vaccinating your partner/relative or friend against disease.

Both men and women benefit enormously if they have loving partners. And there are no side effects. Yet doctors and charities (most of whom are heavily indebted to drug companies) refuse to acknowledge the link between love and health. Many, astonishingly and almost unbelievably, still even seem to reject the idea that there is a link between stress and heart disease. 'There is insufficient evidence to say stress, depression or isolation are main risk factors for heart disease,' a spokeswoman for a heart charity was recently quoted as saying.

Love is a better cure than drugs or surgery. But where's the profit?

42

Any doctor (or other health professional) who confidently tells you what is going to happen to you in a year's time should be sitting on the end of the pier with a scarf around his head and an upturned goldfish bowl on the table in front of him. He should not be practising medicine.

43

Doctors over-diagnose and put unnecessary labels on patients.

44

There is no doubt that some allergy problems (such as asthma) are increasing in their incidence. One reason is that our immune systems have evolved in order to fight infections and we need to be exposed to infections early in life in order to keep them working properly. However, our over-hygienic domestic lifestyle has reduced our natural exposure to mild infections and has, in consequence, sensitised our immune systems which are, as a result, constantly looking for trouble and attacking innocuous aliens such as house dust. Evidence for this comes from research which shows that children who grow up on farms have fewer allergies than children who grow up in towns. This may, it seems, be linked to the number of bugs a child on a farm is likely to encounter. Scientists at Zurich Children's Hospital found two genes which are activated by bacterial infection, and which help to push the immune system away from the direction which causes allergic responses. Both these genes are more active in children who are brought up on farms.

Another problem is undoubtedly the fact that the air in most homes (and schools and offices) is thick with chemical sprays. Air fresheners, oven cleaners, furniture polishes, carpet fresheners and numerous other products contain chemicals which are known to cause asthma. These products are widely used. The result has been a steady and fairly dramatic increase in the incidence of autoimmune disease.

And many vaccines make things worse by reducing the general incidence of childhood infections.

Doctors rarely consider these causes when confronted with a wheezing patient. Encouraged by the drug companies their usual response is to prescribe a powerful new drug. They will often warn the patient (and, if the patient is a child, his or her parents) that drug therapy will be needed for life. The drug companies will have acquired yet another profitable consumer. In the long run, however, there is little doubt that in many cases the drug prescribed will do far more harm than the original symptoms.

45

In the UK there are officially over 500,000 patients suffering from asthma. Some of the drugs used to control asthma can and do kill. If all 500,000 patients really did have asthma then the risk would, of course, be worth taking. But they don't. My guess is that of the 500,000 officially diagnosed, and treated, as asthmatics only a tenth, 50,000 or so, are real asthma sufferers. The other 450,000 have had an occasional wheeze, probably caused by a localised and short-lived chemical allergy but have, nevertheless, been put on long-term treatment.

46

Most doctors think they are more competent than they are. The best doctor is the one who knows that he doesn't know very much.

47

Here's a list of ten diseases for which drugs are over-prescribed. Many of the drug groups on this list are so over-prescribed that they cause more illness than they treat.

1. Osteoporosis
There are three big myths about osteoporosis. The first is that it is a disease which largely affects women. The second is that it is a consequence of the menopause. The third is that the condition can be prevented and/or cured by swallowing calcium. These are marketing tricks established by the drug industry to sell their

products. Osteoporosis is a twenty-first century lifestyle disease best avoided (and conquered) by avoiding tobacco and animal protein (meat), by taking regular, gentle exercise, by avoiding an excessive alcohol intake and by keeping the salt intake down. Too much dieting should also be avoided.

2. Menopause

Millions of women attempt to deal with their menopause by taking hormone replacement therapy. The dangers of this usually unnecessary treatment have been widely documented. Women didn't suffer from the menopause until drug companies recognised it as a marketing opportunity.

3. Asthma

As I have already explained, asthma is now one of the most over-diagnosed diseases. Drug companies have successfully trained doctors and nurses to diagnose asthma on a single wheeze and to initiate lifelong drug therapy. Many drugs and inhalers prescribed for asthma are potentially dangerous. If the patient had asthma the risks would probably be worthwhile. Since the patient for whom the drugs and inhalers have been prescribed probably does not have asthma at all the risks are definitely not worthwhile.

4. Depression

I have little doubt that many of the patients officially diagnosed as suffering from depression would probably be more accurately described as being 'unhappy'. To mix together those suffering from endogenous clinical depression (and needing complex and sometimes dangerous therapy) and those suffering from lifestyle disappointment, crises and stress (and needing advice, help and maybe therapy but advice, help and therapy of an entirely different kind) is absurd, illogical and patently cruel. It is done, quite deliberately by the combined efforts of drug companies which are desperate to sell more of their potent pharmacological compounds and doctors whose debt and allegiance to the pharmaceutical companies far exceeds their perceived debts and allegiance to their patients. Drug companies have successfully encouraged general practitioners to diagnose depression in anyone who doesn't feel entirely happy. Since few of us are entirely happy all the time the official incidence of depression has rocketed in recent years. The drugs prescribed for depression are often exceedingly dangerous and the list of side effects associated with some of the most popularly prescribed products is scary.

5. High blood pressure

Traditionally, high blood pressure has always been over-diagnosed — largely because doctors tend to forget that patients can be nervous when having their blood pressure taken. The condition can, in many patients, be effectively controlled by a mixture of diet, exercise and stress control but doctors tend to find it easier to hand over a prescription. Once a patient has been diagnosed as suffering from high blood pressure, and has been started on medication, the chances are high that the treatment will continue for the rest of the patient's life. Drug companies make huge amounts of money out of pills which were never needed and which, in the long run, do far more harm than good.

6. Arthritis

Arthritis is undoubtedly one of the commonest diseases of middle age and old age. But although it may be painful and disruptive it is not usually life-threatening and can often be managed very effectively by a combination of lifestyle changes. For example, the impact of rheumatoid arthritis can be dramatically reduced if the patient adopts a vegetarian diet. Despite this the usual medical approach is to hand out a prescription — often for an expensive drug which is nowhere near as safe as soluble aspirin and nowhere near as effective either.

7. Obesity

It has become politically incorrect to point out that most people who become grossly obese do so because they eat too much food. Instead the obese are allowed, and even encouraged, to regard themselves as suffering from some sort of illness and are offered treatment of some kind to help them deal with their problem. Inevitably, if no changes are made to eating habits, any weight loss which takes place is quickly reversed. (It is often claimed that stick thin models endanger the health of young girls by encouraging them to stay too thin. Far more damage is done by fat celebrities who revel in their obesity. A quick look around any High Street will reveal that the number of vastly overweight teenage girls is much greater than the number of dangerously underweight teenage girls. The number of diseases associated with obesity is legion.)

8. Tranquillisers

It has been known since 1961 that benzodiazepine drugs are addictive. I first described the problem in 1973 — and predicted that benzodiazepine addiction would be a massive problem within a few years. In the mid 1980s I estimated that there were three million benzodiazepine addicts in Britain alone. And yet even today there are still doctors who are handing out prescriptions for benzodiazepines and who insist that these drugs are perfectly safe, are not addictive and can be taken — and stopped — without any worry. At least

99% of the patients who are given these drugs do not need them and would be better off without them.

9. Maturity onset diabetes (type II diabetes)
Type II diabetes is as near as it is possible to get to an optional disease. Many people who have it could recover if they chose to change their eating habits. Doctors should know this but, bizarrely, they usually just reach for the prescription pad and write out a prescription for a potentially hazardous drug. Once again the drug companies are the only winners.

10. Antibiotics
The rise in the incidence of antibiotic-resistant organisms is due partly to the widespread use of antibiotics by farmers (who recklessly give it to their animals to help speed muscle growth) and partly due to doctors over-prescribing the drugs. Antibiotics are of no value in the treatment of viral infections and yet thousands of doctors regularly hand out prescriptions for antibiotics to patients suffering from influenza (a viral infection).

48
Patients who know more about their illness than their doctor always survive longer than patients who know nothing and who leave everything to the professionals.

49
When your doctor hands you a packet of pills to 'save you the price of a prescription and a trip to the pharmacy', you are probably being used as a guinea pig and helping to test a new drug.

50
Think very carefully before taking a drug that could cause more problems than are caused by the disease

you've already got. Always be cautious about taking drugs if your symptoms are merely irritating and you visited the doctor primarily to make sure that your symptoms didn't denote the onset of something life-threatening. If your doctor prescribes for you ask him if the drugs are really necessary. Ask also what is likely to happen if you don't take the drugs.

This is true of all treatments, not just drugs. If you get killed by a drug that might have saved your life (and you would have died anyway) then taking the drug was an acceptable risk. But if you are killed by a drug which you were taking for something mild and merely uncomfortable, that's a real pain and when you're dead you'll probably never forgive yourself.

51

The mortality rate for a gastric bypass operation widely recommended to help overweight people slim down is 1 in 200.

That means that out of every 200 perfectly healthy but overweight people who have the operation electively one will die. Is that acceptable? I don't think so. Overweight is, it is perfectly true, a major cause of illness. But surgery isn't by any means the only way to lose excess weight. It is, however, the most dangerous.

52

The drug companies are in the business of prolonging illness not curing it. They would be richer if everyone was ill all the time. Indeed, drug company marketing programmes are designed to persuade more and more people that they are ill all the time. For a drug company the idea of nirvana is a world where everyone is always ill and permanently on medication.

The aims and purposes of drug companies are understandable. They exist to make money. That's all.

This purpose does not fit comfortably with that of the medical profession — which exists primarily to diagnose, heal and care for patients. Earning money is important (without it doctors would starve to death) but it is not the primary motive and should not govern the individual doctor's actions, or the attitudes and priorities of the profession as a whole.

In theory the industry and the profession are separate entities, coming together only in that the former manufactures products used by the latter.

But in practice the medical profession and the drug industry have become so closely linked that their aims have become mixed. Many of the doctors who write articles or give lectures about new drugs have received so much funding from drug companies (as consulting fees, grants, bonuses, share options etc.) that their independence has been permanently compromised. Around the world, many medical organisations which exist to evaluate new drugs consist of doctors whose independence must be questioned because of their close financial links with the drug industry.

Things have got so bad that I very much doubt if there is any important medical organisation or committee which is not controlled by doctors whose independence has been totally compromised by their personal financial links to the drug industry.

Over the years I have been widely vilified by leaders of the medical profession for daring to criticise the pharmaceutical industry. To many doctors, criticising the drug industry is on a par with criticising the church or the royal family. The medical profession has, in practice, been little more than an extended marketing arm for the drug industry for several decades.

53

There is now a considerable amount of evidence to show that (with the necessary help of doctors) the multi-billion pound global drug industry frequently manipulates the results of drug trials and withholds inconvenient information which might threaten its profits — even when withholding that information endangers the lives of patients.

The *Journal of the American Medical Association* has published evidence showing that 38% of truly independent studies investigating new drugs reach 'unfavourable' conclusions whereas just 5% of the trials funded by the pharmaceutical industry show that drugs are of no value. Gosh. How could that happen.

54

Of all the bad things the drug industry has done (and a list would fill this book and another eleven volumes like it) the worst must surely be the way they have corrupted the entire medical establishment.

Not that the blame should be laid on one party. You can't be corrupted unless you want to be.

55

Despite extravagant claims to the contrary (largely from the self-serving cancer industry) the incidence of cancer hasn't fallen in recent years. Indeed, the incidence of cancer among children is rising fast. Between the 1970s and 1990s it rose 1 per cent a year for children and 1.5% a year for teenagers. The much publicised efforts of governments and the cancer industry have had a negative effect — they have made things worse.

I'm not surprised by this.

Indeed, it is my belief that cancer charities don't want to see cancer beaten. It is, after all, in their interests for cancer to kill more people. If cancer kills

lots of people the cancer industry will receive lots of
money from worried citizens.

56

When you go to the doctor for help and treatment you
probably assume that once he has decided what is
wrong with you the doctor will automatically give you
a treatment that is quite specific for your disease.

Nothing could be further from the truth.

With a very few exceptions there are no certainties
in medicine. What you will get will depend more on
chance and your doctor's personal prejudices than on
science.

This problem isn't a new one, of course.

In the preface to *The Doctor's Dilemma* playwright
George Bernard Shaw pointed out that during the first
great epidemic of influenza which developed towards
the end of the nineteenth century, a London evening
newspaper sent a journalist posing as a patient to all the
great consultants of the day.

The newspaper then published details of the advice
and prescriptions offered by the consultants.

The whole proceeding was, almost inevitably,
passionately denounced by the medical journals as an
unforgivable breach of confidence, but the result was
nevertheless fascinating: despite the fact that the
journalist had complained of exactly the same
symptoms to all the physicians, the advice and the
prescriptions that were offered were all different.

Nothing has changed.

Even in these days of apparently high technology
medicine there are many — almost endless —
variations in the treatments preferred by different
doctors.

Doctors offer different prescriptions for exactly the
same symptoms, they keep patients in hospital for

vastly different lengths of time, and they perform different operations on patients with apparently identical problems.

There are, it seems, no certainties in medicine. For example, the treatment a patient with cancer gets (whether she has surgery or is given pills) depends largely on which doctor she sees. As one doctor put it rather concisely your treatment (and possibly your future) depends entirely on which way you turn at the end of the hospital corridor. Go left and you will end up having a six hour operation. Go right and you'll go home with a prescription for pills.

There is, indeed, ample evidence now available to show that the type of treatment a patient gets when he visits a doctor will depend not so much on the symptoms he describes but on the doctor he consults.

So, for example, consider what happened when 430 family doctors were asked to explain how they would treat a 35-year-old accountant complaining of backache brought on by digging in his garden.

The 'case history' was deliberately made fairly precise.

However, despite this precision the recommended treatments varied enormously.

Less than a quarter of the doctors said that they would definitely prescribe a painkiller. Nearly ten per cent said that they hardly ever prescribed a painkiller in such circumstances. Eight per cent of the doctors said they might refer the patient to hospital but fifty two percent said that they never referred such patients to hospital. Forty eight per cent said that they usually advised bed rest for up to one week while eight per cent said that they usually advised bed rest for between one and four weeks.

Around ten per cent of the doctors said that there was a good chance that they would refer the patient to an osteopath but the other ninety per cent said that they hardly ever, or never, referred patients to osteopaths.

Going to a general practitioner really is something of a lottery.

Another survey, involving 700 general practitioners, showed that twelve per cent of family doctors might be willing to prescribe a sleeping tablet without even seeing the patient involved. Over half the general practitioners confessed that they would prescribe a cough medicine without seeing a patient and nearly two thirds of the doctors said that they might prescribe an antacid without a patient needing to come into the surgery.

A third survey of over 400 doctors showed that some doctors never provide their patients with any contraceptive advice at all.

Visit three doctors with symptoms of cystitis.

One will give you an antibiotic for five days. One will give you an antibiotic for seven days. And one will give you an antibiotic for ten days. They are all guessing.

Despite all these variations in the type of treatment offered, most doctors in practice seem to be convinced that their treatment methods are beyond question.

Many general practitioners and hospital doctors announce their decisions as though they are carved on stone.

But on the basis of the evidence it seems that most decisions about how patients should be treated are based on nothing more scientific than guesswork, personal experience, intuition and prejudice. And fashion.

57

If there is a high-tech and a low-tech way of doing things, doctors will choose the high-tech approach even if it is less effective and more dangerous.

58

The majority of doctors don't have the time, training or knowledge to help patients suffering from mental illness. They understand very little about the way in which psychological health can and should be managed.

59

According to the World Health Organisation (WHO) depression is now the single commonest cause of disability throughout the world. The WHO claims that 20% of the entire world's population (one in every five of us) is disabled by depression. And that's just depression.

The official figures for other aspects of mental illness, such as anxiety, make equally horrifying reading. One in ten Americans now has or has had a classifiable anxiety disorder. Over two million people in the UK suffer from obsessive compulsive disorder.

Mental illness has (literally) replaced unemployment as Britain's biggest social problem. The biggest single cause of misery in modern western society is not poverty but mental illness.

And around the world the incidence of suicide is increasing rapidly. For example, the incidence of suicide by young men in the UK increased by 175% in the two decades between 1985 and 2005.

There is no doubt that mental illness is on the rise and is one of the most significant and underestimated health problems of our time. And there is no doubt that doctors are poorly trained to deal with these problems, having very little idea about how they are caused and no idea what to do about them.

60

The slightly surprising truth is that human beings now show the same signs of illness as captive zoo animals.

Visit a zoo and watch the animals and you will often see many signs of neurotic behaviour. The polar bears may be swimming round and round in circles. The chimpanzees may be sitting morosely; attempting to amuse themselves by abusing the human spectators. Other animals will have torn out their own fur. Some will eat too much and become obese; succumbing, perhaps, to the temptations offered by the junk food thrown by visitors. Others will eat too little. Many simply sit and stare into space: clearly depressed.

Humans suffer the same diseases. We develop neuroses. We constantly find new ways to abuse ourselves. We develop eating disorders and we acquire addictions.

The problem is that our modern cities are zoos for people. We live as captive animals, pacing around in our cages. Our cities are crowded but millions suffer from loneliness. We have sophisticated communications technology all around us and yet millions hardly ever communicate with other human beings. Countless numbers of people are spiritually empty and suffering as a result.

61

Many people bottle things up because they have no one with whom they can share their problems. New laws removing privacy and confidentiality mean that none of us can expect our conversations with our doctors, lawyers, bank managers, accountants or other advisers to be treated as confidential.

62

Three quarters of the people suffering from depression and other serious mental illness receive little or no effective treatment. The doctor's usual solution is to reach for his prescription pad and write out yet another prescription for yet another anti-depressant or tranquilliser. Occasionally, these drugs might help. Quite often they make things worse. The only consistent winner from this pharmacological solution is the pharmaceutical industry.

63

Is it a coincidence that the quality of medical care has deteriorated over the same period that politicians have forced medical schools to favour female applicants? This egregious example of positive discrimination was introduced because there were more male doctors than female doctors. This was considered politically unacceptable. The result has been that poorly-qualified and poorly-motivated female applicants have taken precedence over well-qualified and well-motivated male applicants. Patients have been the losers. (And the sting in the tail is that many newly-qualified women doctors choose to work part-time, if at all. This is one of the reasons for the chronic shortage of doctors.)

64

Some doctors and nurses are less competent and more stupid than you could possibly imagine them to be.

65

One of the most stupid things doctors do is to give tranquillisers (or, just as daft, anti-depressants) to people who are going through a bereavement.

Grieving, though inevitably painful, is a natural and essential part of bereavement. Tranquillisers do not deal with or banish any of the emotional traumas associated with the loss of a loved one. They merely cover up the sadness and sorrow and numb the mind — acting solely as an anaesthetic rather than as a therapy. The sadness and the pain will remain buried for as long as the tranquillisers are taken. When the pills are stopped the buried sorrow will emerge.

When someone who has been recently bereaved shows signs of sadness they, and those close to them, naturally recognise the source of the sorrow. The tears and the sadness will attract sympathy and understanding which can ease the whole process of mourning.

But when someone who has been bereaved is given a tranquilliser (or a sleeping tablet) the process of mourning is put on ice and delayed until the tablets are stopped. When the drugs are taken away the underlying emotional trauma — which has been merely buried rather than healed — will re-emerge. However, since it may be many months or years since the bereavement which originally inspired those natural (and to a large extent healthy) feelings neither the individual patient nor those around him or her will associate the symptoms being exhibited with something which happened a long time ago. The patient will cry and feel sad but will not know why. And, because there is no obvious cause for the tears and the sadness, those around will find it difficult to understand what is going on.

66

I've written widely and for many years about drug addiction. When I did the research for my books *The Drugs Myth*, *Addicts and Addictions* and *Life Without Tranquillisers* I talked to a good many experts who deal every day with drug addicts.

Based on the advice I was given I came to the conclusion that the six most addictive drugs — in the order of their addictiveness — are:

1. Benzodiazepines
2. Alcohol
3. Tobacco
4. Marijuana
5. Heroin
6. Cocaine

I suspect that lots of people who don't know anything much about drug addiction would find the order of the drugs on that list rather startling. But the truth is that the nonsense we're fed in the movies and by self-serving heroin and cocaine addicts is piffle. The most horrendously addictive drugs in the world are benzodiazepines.

67
Doctors who fail to question everything they are taught and told must invariably do more harm than good.

68
Just because the medical establishment (masquerading as perceived wisdom) says that something is true, doesn't mean that it is true. Indeed, the chances are high that the opposite is true.

69
Medicine only progresses through observation. Sadly, too few doctors and nurses bother to look. And most of those who take the time to look don't see.

Coleman's 6th Law Of Medicine

Hospitals are not suitable places for sick people. If you must go into one, you should get out as quickly as you can.

1

Before the industrial age, hospitals were built like cathedrals in order to lift the soul and ease the mind. Hospitals were decorated with carvings, works of art, flowers and perfumes. Modern hospitals are built with no regard for the spirit, eye or soul. They are bare, more like prisons than temples, designed to concentrate the mind on pain, fear and death. Where there are windows they are positioned in such a way that patients can't see out of them (though even if they could they probably wouldn't be able to see anything more enthralling than the refuse bins or the air-conditioning units).

2

One of the reasons why hospitals are no longer suitable for sick people is the fact that ambitious modern nurses want to administer rather than nurse.

In the dark old days nurses were hired and trained to nurse. Aspiring nurses (mostly but not exclusively female) were inspired by the desire to tend and to heal. Nursing was a noble profession. Caring was the key word. The most powerful jobs in the profession were occupied by ward sisters and matrons — all of whom still had close, daily contact with patients.

Sadly, today's career structure means that nurses whose desire to nurse is accompanied by even the slightest ambition must quickly move up the ladder to a point where they spend very little time or, more probably, no time at all with patients. Nurses used to be trained on the wards. Today nurses are often trained in colleges — far removed from real life patients. Many senior nurses now spend their days closeted in their offices, staring at computer screens and filling in assessment forms. Many seem to regard themselves as above what they see as the menial tasks of nursing. They leave the hands-on work to untrained staff. The introduction of degrees for nurses has turned a fundamentally practical profession into one with entirely spurious academic ambitions. The modern career structure for nurses has taken the best nurses away from patients; it was driven by a patronising and entirely inaccurate concept (that nursing is demeaning).

Today, many nurses go into the profession attracted not by the desire to tend but by the salaries, perks, authority and career structure which will, they know, take them away from practical work. The system is designed to attract exactly the wrong people into nursing.

The actual hands-on nursing is done, very largely, by junior staff.

This is, without a doubt, one of the reasons why modern hospitals are so bad and it is the reason why serious hospital infections are now endemic; it is why nurses are too often rude and uncaring to patients and why, in so many hospitals, clusters of nurses are more likely to be found having meetings (more appropriately called coffee-breaks) than actually helping patients.

Time and time again patients report that nurses won't lift them up the bed (it has been reported that some hospitals have posters with the slogan 'Nurses are not weight lifters' on their walls), won't help feed them, won't bring bedpans, won't change beds, won't do anything for patients in pain or distress and won't respond when the call button is pressed. They will not, in short, do any of the things that nurses are traditionally supposed to do. They are not interested in soothing or healing or helping because they have become career administrators with aspirations and ambitions.

In many hospitals it is the patients who can get out of bed who end up doing all the nursing work.

Stop a nurse in a modern hospital and ask her where such and such a patient can be found or how he or she is progressing and you will probably be met with a glazed, disinterested look. They don't know and they don't much care.

3

Do hospitals need more nurses?

I suspect that most do not.

But hospitals do need the nurses they've got to work harder. My observations (and those of dozens of others) confirm that many nurses seem to spend large parts of their day sitting around gossiping.

4

Hospital staff are constantly complaining about the number of assaults they suffer at the hands of aggrieved patients and relatives. The latest figures show that nearly a third of hospital staff members claim to have been assaulted at some time during their employment. (Much of the abuse consists of complaints and verbal signs of irritation rather than physical violence or threats of physical violence but, rather inevitably perhaps, many staff members are so distressed and traumatised by a little light verbal abuse that they have to take time off work.)

To be honest I'm surprised that the figure is as low as at is. From what I've seen of hospitals in recent years I can only say that the unabused staff members are living charmed lives.

If nurses and other hospital staff members want to stop the assaults they should change their attitude and alter the way they treat and care for patients.

In the United Kingdom a recent survey of National Health Service employees working in hospitals showed that only 44% thought that they would be happy with the standard of care provided if they were patients in their own hospitals.

That really says it all, doesn't it?

5

Modern hospitals tend to be bureaucratic and dangerously overstaffed. Billions of pounds are wasted on salaries, expenses and pensions for unnecessary administrators. Those excess administrators are soaking up so much money that they are indirectly responsible for thousands of deaths.

A spokesman for one hospital which had spent £1,000,000 more than its budget allowed said that the hospital was 'thinking' about what to do (suggesting that the 'hospital' has an identity and a brain and makes its own decisions enables the administrators to avoid taking responsibility) and that what had happened was no one's fault (see what I mean about avoiding responsibility). She said that the hospital was considering selling some equipment or closing some beds in order to deal with its debts. The hospital was not, of course, contemplating getting rid of any of the administrators whose incompetence had led to the problem.

Most administrators seem to believe that hospitals would be much more efficient and cost effective if there were no patients at all. I am sure that they are right.

Signs of administrators at work are everywhere. For example, it is the fashion these days to put carpets on hospital corridors. Naturally, this is dangerously unhealthy (since carpets are far more difficult to clean than other forms of flooring) but at least it means that administrators are not disturbed by the noise of patients being wheeled about.

6

Today Britain's National Health Service employs 1.4 million people. There are 200,000 more employees in the NHS than there were nine years ago. But there are less people actually caring for patients. The number of administrators has grown to exceed both the number of nurses and the number of beds. How, in the name of Hippocrates, can a hospital need more administrators than nurses or more administrators than beds?

7

The present system ensures that the nurses who run hospitals, who make the rules and who provide the 'leadership' are the ones who are least capable of, and least interested in, working directly with patients.

The nurses who run our hospitals are the ones who are least interested in the art of caring, least passionate about nursing as an art and most anxious to climb up the career ladder by exhibiting their prowess at managing meetings, mastering the double-speak that has invaded hospitals and 'giving good mouth'. Nursing lost its way when it became impossible for a nurse to rise in the hierarchy without becoming an administrator. Nursing went wrong when nurses started collecting diplomas and degrees. How can you have a degree in caring?

A few decades ago patients were cared for in hospitals which were run by matrons and ward sisters — nurses who still knew how to turn a patient, make a bed and empty a bedpan. Many patients cannot, of course, remember how efficient hospitals were in those days and so, because they don't know what to expect or what to look for, they think they are being well looked after. Most people have low expectations, are inherently grateful for anything that is done for them, are frightened and don't know what to look for. (This is the only possible explanation for those letters to local newspapers extolling the virtues of the local hospital.) These days the brigades of fat-bottomed nurses who 'administer' our hospitals are too self-important even to look at patients, let alone speak to them. You can occasionally spot these nursing administrators darting along the corridors, eyes averted lest they accidentally soil their vision with the sight of someone in pyjamas or a nightdress. Most of the time these nursing harridans lie hidden behind office doors, planning their career progress. Many of them seem grossly obese — a consequence no doubt of doing too little work and spending too much time munching chocolates and biscuits.

8

There is very little continuity of nursing care in modern hospitals. Patients are lucky if they ever see the same nurse twice. Those who are left at the dirty end of the profession, wander around almost uninterested in their work. Often slovenly and untidy, they do not seem to care for their patients at all. Visit a modern hospital ward and it is frequently difficult, if not impossible, to tell who is in charge. The modern nurses' office (or 'station') will usually be positioned in a spot where the nurses can hide away from the patients to make their phone calls, eat their chocolates and gossip. Inevitably, if the patients cannot see the nurses, the converse is also true: the nurses cannot see the patients. Calls for help or bedpans go unnoticed.

9

In many countries, doctors (both in general practice and in hospitals) are now working strictly limited hours. Many general practitioners no longer provide the 24 hour, 365 day service which was an integral part of family practice just a few years ago. The modern general practitioner works the sort of hours usually associated with school teachers, librarians and accountants. Many hospital doctors now work only short, fixed weeks. It is rare to see a doctor (or a physiotherapist or, indeed, anyone else who isn't a patient or a visitor) in a hospital at weekends these days. Patients are left lying in bed all weekend. No one, it seems, has heard of deep vein thromboses or pressure sores.

10

One result of the shortage of doctors has been that nurses have been given the right to prescribe and to perform surgery — and to take on these responsibilities without any medical supervision and without the sort of training required for doctors. To the problem of bad prescribing by doctors has now been added the problem bad prescribing by nurses. Most nurses (like most doctors) know very little about the drugs they prescribe and know next to nothing about side effects.

Patients need fewer — not more — people handing out prescriptions.

11

Infections are now a major killer in our hospitals. Thousands of patients are killed by antibiotic-resistant infections. The methicillin resistant staphylococcus aureus (MRSA) bug kills and seriously injures thousands of people every year. Hygiene standards are appalling. Wards are often filthy and nurses and doctors often fail to wash their bloody, bug-stained hands when moving from one patient to another. Hygiene in hospitals is just a word (which most members of staff probably cannot even spell).

Visit a hospital and watch the cleaners at work: you'll see them slide a mop down the centre of the ward (this is known in the mop wielding business as 'taking the mop for a walk') but leave the space under the beds or around the lockers unswept. The cleaners then wander off into their staff room for a tea break.

Staggeringly, the same people who clean the ward then serve patients their food. No one seems to see anything odd in this. The cleaners do not, of course, wash their hands between these two activities. Cleaning staff (sorry, I think they now have to be called 'housekeepers') do not appear to have been told that they too must obey the basic rules of hygiene. I have seen a cleaner go into a private room containing a patient with MRSA without bothering to put on mask, gloves or gown.

The Government would save far more lives if it took down speed cameras and, instead, put up cameras in hospitals to check that nurses, cleaners and doctors washed their hands properly. Such a simple action would save billions of pounds and thousands of lives a year. Nurses who are spotted moving from patient to patient without washing their hands should be fired and banned from ever working in health care again.

12

The separation of authority from responsibility means that doctors are no longer in charge of what happens to their patients. Doctors work in teams (as equal members alongside such dross as social workers) led by administrators. Today, it is the administrators who are in charge. And administrators are, it seems, unsackable. Whenever a hospital runs short of money it is the facilities for patients which are cut — never the number of overpaid, underworked administrators. It is not difficult to sustain the belief that modern hospitals and health centres are run for employees in general, and administrators in particular, rather than for patients.

13

Dignity is not a word which the modern nurse understands.

Not, at least, when applied to patients. Many hospitals still have mixed wards — with male and female patients forced to abandon their natural dignity in the interests of hospital economy (so that the administrators can take yet another huge pay rise). In Britain the Government has repeatedly promised to make sure that mixed wards are done away with. Inevitably this promise, like most of the others governments make, has been forgotten. Patients (particularly elderly ones) are talked to as if they were slightly backward children; invariably being addressed by their first names rather than being given the respect and dignity afforded by the prefix Mr or Mrs. In many hospitals, patients are given revealing little gowns to wear. These hide nothing from general view but patients are instructed that they must be worn without underwear. Patrons in the seediest type of nightclub would be arrested if they wore such revealing attire.

14

Much of the medical establishment still steadfastly and stubbornly refuses to acknowledge that 'alternative' or 'complementary' medical techniques have anything to offer. Gentle therapies, and gentle practitioners, are deliberately demonised by the drug industry controlled medical establishment.

15

The food in hospitals is diabolical and contributes enormously to the death rate among patients. It is, for example, quite absurd that hospitals should continue to serve meat dishes to patients. Since the evidence linking meat to cancer is just as convincing as that linking tobacco to cancer, it would make as much sense for nurses to walk around the wards handing out cigarettes.

16

A study of 1,203 patients who had heart attacks showed that staying at home may be safer than going into hospital. The patients in the trial were allocated at random either to a hospital bed or to staying at home. The authors of the paper reported that the mortality rates for the two groups were similar. Whatever advantage patients might have had through going into hospital and being surrounded by machines, doctors and nurses, was matched by the hazards of going into hospital.

17

Hospitals are dangerous places for several reasons but the most important is the fact that you are more likely to catch a serious, life-threatening infection in hospital than anywhere else. The great danger is, of course, that you may catch an MRSA infection. (MRSA is a superbug which is resistant to most if not all available antibiotics.) Such infections were predictable (I predicted their development in 1977 in a book called *Paper Doctors*) and are avoidable (I explained how they could best be avoided in the same book) but as a result of worsening hospital hygiene (neither doctors nor nurses bother to wash their hands anywhere near often enough) and the overuse of antibiotics, MRSA is now a significant health threat in hospitals.

The MRSA problem has two causes. First, the over-prescribing of antibiotics by doctors. Second, the fact that farmers give their animals regular doses of antibiotics in order to keep them healthy and to increase their weight gain.

The e.coli 0157 bug which causes so many problems — bloody diarrhoea for the lucky and kidney failure for the not so lucky — first emerged in intensively reared cattle and is probably a result of the excessive use of antibiotics as growth promoters and prophylactics. The long-term use of antibiotics harms the normal intestinal microorganisms which keep e.coli 0157 in check. Normally animals can rebalance their intestinal microflora in order to get rid of the deadly e.coli variation but they cannot do this when they are confined in modern factory farms.

The result of this reckless over-use of antibiotics by doctors and farmers is that most of the diseases which we thought we had eradicated have come back, stronger than ever and more resistant to the drugs available to us.

We are on a downhill slope that is getting steeper by the day. Our expectations are unrealistic and our approach is faulty. Hospitals in the UK are the worst in the world for this particular problem and British patients in National Health Service hospitals are 40 times as likely to get an MRSA infection as are patients in hospitals in other European countries. Hospital staff seem unconcerned at this even though every incidence of MRSA infection is straightforward evidence of nursing incompetence. Even medical records, pens and computer keyboards are now known to be infected with MRSA. In many hospitals nurses are not given enough uniforms to be able to change daily. Some hospitals have no changing facilities and so nurses go home in their uniforms (taking bugs with them). Most hospitals don't launder uniforms and so nurses have to put their uniforms in with the family wash — usually at a temperature which will not destroy the bugs.

If the spread of the infection is to be halted hospitals will need to be closed down one by one and thoroughly cleaned before being re-opened.

Progress might speed up a little if a few dozen doctors, nurses and administrators were imprisoned for manslaughter. (It's difficult to see why they shouldn't be. Running or working in a dirty hospital is just as much a crime as driving while drunk or under the influence of drugs.)

Meanwhile, things are likely to continue to get worse. One British hospital where superbug infections doubled in just two years admitted that its cleaners mop under patients' beds only once a week. The hospital's chief executive admitted that only about 30% of hospital floor space is cleaned but seemed proud of the fact that some areas of the hospital were cleaned on a daily basis.

It is ignorance and arrogance like this which has led to the MRSA epidemic.

Hospital administrators (the ones who make all the decisions these days) do not seem to understand that patients in hospital are likely to have under-efficient immune systems and, therefore, to be vulnerable to infection.

Keeping hospitals clean isn't difficult. All it needs is regular washing of hands and cleaning of surfaces (and floors) with soap and water. Sadly, most doctors and nurses (and indeed other staff) seem to think that washing their hands or cleaning equipment is beneath them. One former radiologist reports having picked up a probe she needed to use to perform a breast scan and finding a pubic hair still attached to it. It turned out that the previous patient had been a man being scanned for testicular cancer. Most doctors working in modern hospitals regard similar horror stories as too day-to-day to merit note. Surgeons report being telephoned hours after an operation and told that a patient upon whom they had operated had MRSA. And any senior nurse or doctor who does remind a more junior colleague to wash their hands is quite likely to find themselves facing a disciplinary board while the grubby handed member of staff will take nine months sick leave to recover from the stress of being told off.

As if all that wasn't bad enough, you are also more likely to catch a less serious, but debilitating infection in a hospital than you are elsewhere. In some parts of the world hospital food is handled with scant regard for the basic rules of hygiene. It is hardly surprising, therefore, that the risk of contracting an ordinary vomiting and diarrhoea bug in hospital is greater than almost anywhere else. Not even grubby back street cafes can match hospitals when it comes to counting the number of 'customers' brought low by stomach bugs.

18

Once you are in hospital doctors will feel an urge to do things to you. Some of these things will be useful. Many will not. Blood will be removed, X-rays will be taken and other tests performed. There are two risks with having tests done.

The first is the risk inherent in the test itself. Every time a venepuncture is performed there is a risk that you will contract an infection. Every time you have an X-ray you are increasing your chances of developing cancer.

The second is the risk associated with the tendency of doctors to treat test results rather than patients. Many tests produce inaccurate or misleading results and the danger is that doctors will be tempted to assume that the test results imply the existence of pathology you don't have. You may, therefore, be subjected to an operation you don't need or given drugs for no good reason. Operations are potentially dangerous procedures and are best avoided whenever possible.

19

Surgical deaths in the United Kingdom alone are said to number between 20,000 and 30,000 a year. Anaesthesia is a regular cause of serious problems — resulting in thousands of deaths.

Many of the conditions for which the doomed patients entered the operating theatre might not have proved fatal by themselves. In other words those patients were killed by the surgery.

20

The risks associated with routine surgery are not widely understood (and are usually dramatically under-estimated by doctors). Nine out of ten operations are done to improve life rather than save life. This means that 90% of the patients who die as a result of surgery didn't *need* their operations. Little research has been done to find out if all those operations actually do improve the quality of life for the patients who have them.

21

Complex modern medical and surgical treatments often involve ethical dilemmas which are rarely discussed in public. I wonder, for example, how many people know that in order to transplant a heart the organ must still be beating when it is removed from the donor patient.

22

To all this, of course, must be added the fact that 40% of patients given drugs (and how many patients in hospital are not given drugs?) will suffer painful, uncomfortable or potentially fatal side effects.

23

One officially unrecognised danger of going into hospital is that you may starve to death. The food in many hospitals is dire. It lacks nutritional value but is full of saturated fats.

But there is another danger: the real risk that patients who are seriously ill will not receive the food they need — however poor it may be.

I have seen patients in hospital unable to feed themselves who have clearly been slowly starving to death.

The problem is simple.

The staff bring round a meal and place it on the patient's table.

The patient is too ill or too weak to do anything with the meal.

Twenty minutes later the staff come round again, collect up the untouched food and hurry away with an uncaring and thoughtless 'Not hungry today, dear?' tossed over a shoulder.

The patient, increasingly weak and hungry, simply waves a hand in mild protest and then sinks back into the pillows again.

Eventually the patient starves to death. This happens often. Patients in hospital need a relative or friend to feed them if they cannot feed themselves.

24

Hospital patients are rarely given their pills on time. The handing out of drugs is one of the most important activities on a hospital ward. It used to be something that was carried out by the ward sister. These days it is regarded as a chore to be delegated. The senior nursing staff will be far too busy filling in forms (or designing new ones) to bother with anything that involves interacting with patients. The result is that patients rarely get their pills when they should. Drugs don't work as efficiently when given randomly.

25

Patients who need a bedpan will often be left to shout and buzz for help for many minutes. When another patient eventually manages to persuade a nurse or auxiliary to attend it will often be done with poor grace and little or no concern for the patient's feelings. Once the patient is stuck on a bedpan he or she is likely to remain there far longer than is necessary. Once again it will often require the intervention of other patients to attract the attention of a member of staff since for long periods the ward is likely to be unattended while staff members attend meetings or consume yet more coffee.

26

Hospital complaints procedures are designed to protect the hospital from litigation and the staff member from trouble, rather than to protect the patient from abuse or mistreatment. Consequently, there is little or no point in complaining about the quality of care provided in hospitals. The standard official response for hospitals these days is to say that they are improving/updating/reviewing their internal practices and that a full on-going investigation is under way. They repeat this mantra endlessly in the hope and belief that you will eventually drop your complaint and (erroneously) assume that you have had some impact on the way things are done. No individuals employed by the hospital are ever expected to take responsibility for their actions. In our harsh and uncaring modern world, strangers (even ones who are paid to care) will never care as much about your loved one's health and comfort as you do.

27

Hospitals are particularly dangerous places at weekends. The risks of being admitted to hospital at the weekend are quantifiable and scary. You are between 8% and 26% more likely to die if you are admitted to hospital at the weekend than if you are admitted to hospital during the week.

One reason for this is that senior doctors go home, often leaving very junior doctors to look after vast numbers of patients. Theoretically, it should be possible for a junior doctor to call in a consultant. In practice this hardly ever happens, partly because not many young doctors have the courage to pull a senior consultant off the golf course and partly because the senior consultant may have disappeared and be unreachable. In many hospitals this means that a patient may receive no treatment at all over the weekend. But it isn't just doctors who are in short supply. Nurses are scarce too. Senior nurses may disappear completely, leaving relatively junior nurses in charge. Technical staff are likely to be unavailable and equipment will probably be locked up and unusable. While writing this book I read about a teenage boy who died in hospital after collapsing with a brain haemorrhage. Doctors at the large hospital where he was a patient told the boy's mother that he needed an angiogram — an X-ray of blood vessels in his brain — so that they could decide how best they should treat him. But they said that the procedure wasn't available at weekends. Administrators can be blamed for this appalling attitude but doctors must take some responsibility too. They should force the bureaucrats into action.

28

More and more hospitals are now so busy manipulating their figures to make themselves look good that they don't have the time to do things that would actually make things better. So, for example, many hospitals keep their surgical waiting lists short by ensuring that the patients needing relatively simple surgery are treated first. It is obviously quicker to deal with 12 patients requiring surgery that will take 20 minutes than it is to deal with one patient who requires surgery that will take 10 hours. Attempts to disguise the truth seem endlessly Machiavellian. One reader of mine reported to me that after he had had to wait nearly two hours later than his appointment time he complained. The hospital wrote and told him that he was wrong and that he had left the clinic after a 45 minute wait. When my reader produced witnesses disputing this the hospital spokesman wrote back admitting that: '...I have discovered that patients are often booked out or 'departed' from clinics at a time that does not necessarily correspond to the actual time they left the clinic'. Just what sort of problems this could create in the case of a fire or some other crisis it is difficult to imagine.

29

In the United Kingdom the number of senior managers in hospitals has risen every year for decades. In 1951 UK hospitals were managed by 29,021 administrators and clerks. By 2003 the number of administrators had risen to 253,613 so the work was being shared by nearly ten times as many people. The number of domestic staff employed had, during the same period, fallen from 163,660 to 138,238 (explaining, perhaps, why hospitals are getting dirtier and dirtier). In 1953 there were 34.2 hospital beds for every member of the medical staff. Half a century later this had fallen to 2.7 hospital beds for every member of the medical staff. In 1953 there were 467,000 available hospital beds in the NHS. Half a century later there were just 198,000 available hospital beds in NHS hospitals. (The number of inpatient acute hospital beds in the UK is approximately one third the number in the Czech Republic and Slovakia.)

30

The world is, it seems, full of clerks these days. Most of them love to acquire authority but eschew responsibility. And most of them seem to have found jobs in health care where doctors, reluctant to take on paperwork, and not aware that in the 21st century the power goes with the paperwork, have unwittingly left a power vacuum.

31

Hospitals are designed and built around the needs of the staff. To the architects who design hospitals, to the managers who run them, and to the staff who work in them, patients are, it seems, something of a nuisance, without whom everything would run far more smoothly.

If hospitals were designed with the safety and convenience of patients in mind wards would be built in a star shape, with a bed in each point of the star and a nurses' station in the centre of the star. Through one of the points of the star there would be a single entrance to the ward. Individual wards would be attached by short corridors to the points of another, much larger star. The stores and resuscitation equipment would be kept in the centre of this larger star. Specialist departments (such as X-ray units) would be attached to points of the larger star.

This design would provide some privacy for patients, but would make it possible for staff to observe patients at all times. And it would ensure that long journeys along hospital corridors would be banished since no patients would ever be very far from any specialist unit — or, indeed, from another ward. The star shape would make it easy to seal off infected wards. I suspect that staff wouldn't like my design very much for just as it would allow them to keep an eye on patients so it would allow patients to keep an eye on them.

32

The people who work in hospitals (and the people who run them) rarely, if ever, look for ways to reduce the number of errors made. The usual response is to deny that anything untoward has happened at all. This response probably originated as a defence against litigation. But it has become the standard. It is hardly surprising that things are continually getting worse, and that the same mistakes are constantly being repeated. If doctors, nurses and administrators would have the courage to apologise and explain occasionally they would find that their relationship with their patients might be mended and even restored to its former condition. But while doctors, nurses and administrators continue to deny obvious truths the relationship between staff and patients will continue to deteriorate.

33

Hospital staff are too often underworked and lazy. Hospitals are filthy dirty and badly run. Hospitals have too much money but ill-informed, uncaring, self-serving bureaucrats spend it on all the wrong things. If the Gestapo ever gets back on its feet and starts recruiting it will have little difficulty in finding suitable candidates among the administrators working in hospitals.

Sadly, hospitals won't improve because the administrators won't do what they ought to do — sack themselves.

34

Non-emergency (or elective) surgery is always the treatment of last resort.

35

As hospitals become increasingly dangerous places more and more patients will choose to stay at home rather than risk going to hospital. Patients who need to be in hospital (for an operation or an invasive investigation) may choose to convalesce at home.

Would you know how to cope if you had to become a nurse overnight? Every day thousands of men and women find themselves having to cope with an invalid in the house.

Here are some tips that will help make things easier for you if anyone in your family needs looking after at home.

1. Few patients need to stay in bed all day. Unless the doctor has given instructions to the contrary your patient should be able to get up out of bed to bathe and use the toilet. Most patients feel better if they are allowed to get up, watch TV or sit in a chair.

2. If you do have to look after a patient who is going to be bed-bound try and get hold of a hospital-type bed. They are much higher than ordinary beds. Bending over an ordinary divan for more than a few days will soon give you a bad back.

3. Sick rooms get stuffy. Don't be afraid to have a window open. Germs like stale air.

4. Try to change the sheets as often as you can. Crisp, clean bed sheets are wonderful. Powdering with talc helps to prevent the development of bedsores in long-term patients.

5. If your patient needs to take pills keep a chart by the bedside and tick off pills and medicines when they are given. That way you won't be left wondering whether or not you have given the right dose at the right time.

6. Patients often have poor appetites. Try to make food as attractive as possible. Don't put too much on the plate at once. Remember that weak patients are often better off with foods that don't need too much chewing or cutting.

7. If you need help or advice ask your doctor to arrange for a district nurse to call. She should be able

to offer expert, professional advice and maybe lend you useful equipment.

8. To save too many journeys up and down the stairs fill a vacuum flask with an iced drink and keep it by the bedside.

9. Try to fix up some sort of communication system. Even a walking stick that can be banged on the floor is better than nothing.

10. Give your patient things to look forward to. Point out good programmes on the TV or radio. Keep magazines, books, puzzles etc. on one side for really dull moments. And although visitors can be a help remember that too many visitors can be very tiring.

36

Doctors have far more power over administrators than most of them realise. For example, doctors don't use the power of the death. certificate anywhere near enough. When I worked as a general practitioner I quickly discovered that I had complete power over most small-minded bureaucrats. If they wouldn't do what I thought necessary for the care of my patients I would merely point out that if anything happened as a result of their failure to follow my advice (or respond to my request) I would, if the patient died, write their name on the death certificate as a cause of death. For example, I remember an administrator telling me, with great delight, that it would take four months for the system to deliver to me the medical notes relating to a patient who had recently moved to my practice. After using my death certificate ploy I had the medical records on my desk in less than fifteen minutes. If I was in practice these days I would use the same trick to persuade politicians as well as administrators to respond to requests with more compassion and more consideration.

Coleman's 7th Law Of Medicine

There are fashions in medicine just as much as there are fashions in clothes. The difference is that whereas badly conceived fashions in clothes are only likely to embarrass you, ill-conceived fashions in medicine may kill you. The fashions in medicine have, by and large, as much scientific validity as the fashions in the clothes industry.

1

The most obvious fashions in medicine relate to treatments. For example, a couple of centuries ago, enemas, purges and bleedings were all the rage. In 17th century France, Louis XIII had 212 enemas, 215 purges and 47 bleedings in a single year. The Canon of Troyes is reputed to have had a total of 2,190 enemas in a two year period; how he found time to do anything else is difficult to imagine. By the mid 19th century enemas were a little last year's style and bleeding was the in-thing. There was even a posh word for it — doctors who were about to remove blood from their patients would say that they were going to phlebotomize them. Patients would totter into their doctor's surgery, sit down, tuck up their sleeves and ask the doctor to 'draw me a pint of blood'. Bleeding was the universal cure, recommended for most symptoms and ailments. 'Feeling a little under the weather? A little light bleeding should soon put you to rights.' 'Constant headaches? We'll soon have that sorted for you, sir. Just roll up your sleeve.' 'Bit of trouble down below, madam? Not to worry. Slip off your frock and hold your arm out.'

A little later, in the nineteenth century, doctors put their lancets away and started recommending alcohol as the new panacea. Brandy was the favoured remedy in the doctor's pharmacopoeia. People took it for almost everything. And when patients developed delirium tremens the recommended treatment was more alcohol. If things got so bad that the brandy didn't work doctors added a little opium. Those were the days to be ill. Hypochondriacs must have had a wonderful time.

In the years from the 1930s onwards removing tonsils became the fashionable treatment. Tonsils were removed from between a half and three-quarters of all children in the 1930s. This often useless and unnecessary, and always potentially hazardous, operation is less commonly performed these days but in the 1970s over a million such operations were done every year in Britain alone. Doctors used to rip out tonsils on the kitchen table and toss them to the dog. Between 200 and 300 deaths a year were caused by the operation. One suspects that few, if any, of those unfortunate children would have died from tonsillitis.

2

Diseases go in cycles too. In the early 19th century the fashionable diagnosis was 'inflammation'. Then, when patients and doctors tired of that, the new key word was 'debility'. Doctors didn't know terribly much and so their diagnoses, like their treatments, tended to be rather general.

These days patients expect more specific diagnoses and doctors are invariably happy to oblige.

One year everyone will be suffering from asthma. It will be the disease of the moment just as the mini skirt or ripped jeans may drift mysteriously in and out of fashion. Another year arthritis will be the fashionable disease as a drug company persuades journalists to write articles extolling the virtues (and disguising the vices) of its latest product. Depression. Irritable bowel syndrome. Osteoporosis. The cycle is a relatively simple one. The drug company with a new and profitable product to sell (usually designed for some long-term — and therefore immensely profitable — disorder) will send teams of well-trained representatives around to talk to family physicians, give them presents and take them out for expensive luncheons. The sales representatives will be equipped with information showing that the disorder in question is rapidly reaching epidemic proportions, lists of warning symptoms for the doctor to watch out for and information about the drug company's new solution to the problem. Because the product will be new to the market there will probably be very little evidence available about side effects and the sales representative will be accurately able to describe the drug as extremely 'safe'.

Not surprisingly, thousands of family doctors will respond to this hard-sell system by diagnosing more of the disease in question and handing out fistfuls of prescriptions for the recommended product. Older drugs, well-tried, possibly effective and probably safer than the new replacement, will be discarded as out-of-date. After all, their side effects will, over the years, have been well-documented.

As the disease subsequently seems to become more widespread so articles will appear about it in newspapers and magazines, and television pundits will start to talk about it. Every patient who has the appropriate symptoms (however mildly) will be convinced that he or she is suffering from the disease in question.

And the number of prescriptions being written for the new wonder product will soon rocket — pushing up drug company profits dramatically.

Then, a year or so later, patients and doctors alike will become aware of the many side effects associated with the new alleged wonder product and prescribing levels will fall. It is then the turn of some other product and some other disease to take the limelight and some other drug company to enjoy a dramatic boost in its profits.

3

For years now surgeons have been performing unnecessary operations; operations which have done far more harm than good. It is, of course, difficult to be precise about the number of unnecessary operations but in America researchers have concluded that in an average sort of year surgeons working in American hospitals now perform 7.5 million unnecessary surgical procedures, resulting in 37,136 unnecessary deaths and a cost running into hundreds of billions of dollars. (This should be compared with figures for 1974 when there were 2.4 million unnecessary surgical procedures, resulting in 11,900 unnecessary deaths and an annual cost of $3.9 billion.)

The figures for unnecessary surgeries were derived from the USA Congressional Committee on Interstate Foreign Commerce hearings on unnecessary surgery. The Committee found that 17.6% of recommendations for surgery were not necessary and it was the House Subcommittee on Oversight and Investigations which produced the figures I have quoted above.

4

Tonsillectomy may have gone out of fashion (partly because doctors realised at last that the tonsils are actually quite useful) but vast numbers of children still have perfectly healthy appendices ripped out. At the other end of the age spectrum untold millions have had unnecessary surgery for hernias which would have probably never caused serious problems if they had been left alone. Millions of women have had their wombs removed. (In America, one third of women have had a hysterectomy before they reach the menopause.) Many pregnant women deliver their babies via Caesarian section either because this suits the obstetrician's desire to avoid being called from the golf course or because it suits the mother who prefers to have a small hardly visible scar rather than the consequences of vaginal delivery or because it enables the surgeon to charge a fat fee for surplanting nature. Astonishingly around a quarter of babies are delivered this way in America. (Is one in four American mothers really unable to deliver a baby the normal way? In the Netherlands only 8% of babies are delivered by Caesarian section.) Many spinal operations are regarded by independent surgeons as unnecessary and untold thousands of men have had radical but unnecessary treatment for prostate disease (many of them diagnosed through blood tests now known to be of very doubtful value).

5

Surgery often ends up wrecking people's lives, rather than saving them. For example, men subjected to unnecessary prostate surgery may end up impotent or incontinent. If you need an operation (and may die without it) then the risk is undoubtedly worthwhile. If you don't really need an operation then you shouldn't have one. Sadly for patients a lot of surgeons will happily operate on patients whether they need surgery or not. It is, of course, just a coincidence that the surgeon who operates most usually has the biggest car, the smartest holiday villa and the best golf clubs.

6

When an operation is vital and potentially life-saving then the risks are, of course, worth taking. But elective operations performed simply because surgery is what surgeons do (and because no one has bothered to work out whether the advantages outweigh the disadvantages) are illogical and unforgivable.

It was, for example, pointed out some years ago that the mortality risk of elective herniorrhaphy in men over the age of 65 is four times greater than the risk of allowing the hernia to strangulate and require treatment with emergency surgery. In other words if you are a 65-year-old man and you have a hernia, it may well be safer for you to keep your hernia and have it operated upon only if it causes pain and needs emergency attention. Your general health and the nature of your hernia must be considered before an operation is contemplated. Too often the surgeon will see a hernia and just shovel the patient onto the operating table without even bothering to consider the alternatives. Even when the patient is healthy and the surgeon experienced there are many things that can go wrong. Even with caring surgeons and nurses, instruments and swabs are sometimes left inside when the wounds are closed, and wounds may bleed or become infected.

7

Nothing illustrates the uselessness (and danger) of elective surgery more completely than heart surgery. In America, having had at least one coronary artery bypass operation is now as much a sign of success as ownership of a Mercedes limousine. And the operation is growing in popularity around the rest of the world. In Britain, 28,000 coronary artery bypass operations are performed each year — that's around 10% of the people who have had heart attacks.

Many surgeons claim that surgery for heart disease is not elective but vital. But the evidence shows that most of the surgery performed for the treatment of heart disease is entirely unnecessary. Back in 1988 (in a book called *The Health Scandal*) I reported that coronary artery bypass surgery (the commonest procedure performed in cardiac surgery) had been in use for nearly thirty years without anyone trying to find out how patients' everyday lives were affected by the operation. When a survey was eventually done it was found that whereas nearly half of the patients who had the operation had been working right up to the time of surgery, three months after the operation only just over a third of the men were working. And a year after the operation nearly half the patients were still not working. In other words, the operation had little positive effect on patients' lives but did put a good many out of action for some time. There were, of course, a number of patients who died as a result of surgical complications. A bypass operation takes several hours to perform, consumes a good deal of hospital time and professional skill and can be a physically and mentally exhausting experience for a patient and his family. There is a one in thirty risk that a patient undergoing coronary artery bypass surgery will be dead within thirty days of the operation. The mortality rate varies from surgeon to surgeon but it can be as high as 20% and anything up to a quarter of patients having the operation have heart attacks either while on the operating table or shortly afterwards.

And what makes the medical profession's enthusiasm for coronary artery surgery even more bizarre is the fact that patients who have symptoms of heart disease don't need surgery at all but stand a better chance of recovering if they are put on a regime which includes a vegan diet, gentle exercise and relaxation. (I described the utterly convincing evidence for this in my book *How To Stop Your Doctor Killing You,* which was first published in 1996. The chapter is entitled Conquer Heart Disease Without Pills Or Surgery.)

Twenty years ago I found it difficult to avoid the conclusion that any doctor who routinely recommends surgery for patients who show signs or symptoms of heart disease is a homicidal maniac who should be struck off the medical register and locked up.

But doctors continue to recommend elective heart surgery. And surgeons continue to perform heart surgery on patients who could have got better without going into hospital at all. And some surgeons continue to have a far worse record than others. In 2005, for example, it was reported that a heart patient's chance of dying after an operation in a British hospital can be up to seven times higher with some surgeons than with others. Would you visit a hairdresser who was seven times as likely to chop off your ear as the competition?

8

I'm pleased to say that recently the medical profession has begun to look a little critically at heart surgery.

In 2005, *Business Week* magazine quoted an American professor of medicine as saying that bypass surgery 'should have been relegated to the archives 15 years ago'. And the magazine reported that the data from clinical trials shows that except in a minority of patients with severe disease, bypass operations don't prolong life or prevent future heart attacks.

One problem which *Business Week* didn't mention is that if patients have heart surgery and do not change their lifestyles (but continue eating the wrong foods, smoking, taking too much stress and avoiding exercise) then they will need another operation within a few years.

On the other hand patients who adopt the curative lifestyle changes I have described (including regular exercise, a vegan diet and learning to relax) are likely to find that their cure is permanent.

9

It's easy to see why surgeons continue performing heart surgery. (You only have to look at the line up of Mercedes and BMWs in the doctors' car park). Surgeons make their living by operating on people and are, therefore, unlikely to recommend a form of treatment that doesn't involve knives and sutures. But why do physicians and general practitioners continue to recommend patients for operations that are, on balance, more likely to do them harm than good? Could it be that the heart surgery industry — worth an estimated $100 billion a year-is just very good at denying and disguising the truth?

10

The vast majority of medical journalists, who might be expected to criticise unnecessary medical procedures which put patients' lives at risk, know little or nothing of medical matters and are too much in awe of the medical establishment to offer any sort of criticism.

11

Few things illustrate the medical profession's enthusiasm for fashion better than the way that doctors gave credence to the AIDS myth in the 1980s. AIDS was, for a while, the most fashionable disease in history. (Politicians and journalists created the hysteria which surrounded AIDS but it was doctors who gave the disease its false credibility.)

In the 1980s a spokesman for the British Medical Association warned that by 1991 every family in Britain would be touched be AIDS, and attacked me viciously when I quoted evidence supporting a less scary point of view. Other medical establishment groups jumped on the 'AIDS is going to kill us all so give us lots of money to try and find a cure' bandwagon and the official line was defended with unprecedented ferocity and an astonishing amount of self-righteous, sanctimonious venom.

The World Health Organisation forecast that 100 million people might be infected by the year 1990 and the Royal College of Nursing in the UK forecast that one in fifty people in Britain would have the disease by the early 1990s. As far as I know none of these groups has apologised for its absurd scaremongering and none has provided an explanation for the size of its error.

In addition, numerous organisations and individuals who were applying for grants, made dramatic promises of 'miracle breakthroughs' and 'wonder vaccines', probably because they knew that the bigger the promise the larger the grant would probably be.

In the late 1980s and early 1990s I rejected the theory put forward by every scaremongering half-wit eager to jump on the 'AIDS is the biggest plague to hit mankind' bandwagon. For a variety of self-serving reasons which had nothing to do with medicine many scaremongers were claiming that AIDS was a sexually transmitted disease and was likely to wipe out a large proportion of the western world. At the time I was vilified for daring to point out that all the available scientific evidence showed that AIDS was not going to be the plague that killed us all.

The evidence shows that I was right and there is now no doubt that the original predictions for AIDS have all been proved utterly wrong. Because AIDS offers an excellent example of a disease that became fashionable it is worth exploring in a little more detail.

12

Early in 1987 an ex-soldier called Michael Coles, a 42-year-old father of two, picked up a shotgun and blasted his eighteen-year-old son in the back. He then killed his 39-year-old wife before turning the shotgun on himself. The coroner recorded that Mrs Coles had been unlawfully killed and that her husband had committed suicide. Their eighteen-year-old son survived.

Mr Coles took this dreadful step because he thought he had AIDS. He decided to wipe out his family in case he had infected them. And he decided to kill himself to avoid the misery and suffering that he considered inevitable.

In fact he didn't have AIDS at all. He had 'flu. But like millions of other perfectly ordinary healthy individuals, he had been terrified out of his mind by the propaganda from which it was impossible to escape at the time.

Michael Coles, like many others, was convinced that AIDS threatened us all and that it was a common, easily caught, inevitably lethal disease. He had believed what his government had told him, what he had heard on television and what he'd read in the newspapers. The real tragedy is that he, like everyone else, had been conned.

13

In *The Health Scandal* (published in 1988) I wrote that 'from the facts that are available it is clear that AIDS is not going to be the disease that wipes out mankind.'

And I published a true anecdote designed to make it clear why the public image of this disease was so horribly inaccurate.

14

I reported that in early 1987 I had received a telephone call from a researcher for a TV company who had told me that his company was planning a documentary about AIDS.'

'What do you think about AIDS?' he asked me.

I told him that I thought that the threat had been exaggerated by some doctors, a lot of politicians and most journalists. The researcher was silent for a moment or two. I could tell by the silence that he was disappointed. It wasn't quite what he'd hoped to hear.

We're planning a major documentary,' he said. 'We want to cover all the angles. Haven't you got anything new to say about AIDS?'

'I don't think AIDS is a plague that threatens mankind,' I insisted.

I then pointed out that I believed that the evidence about AIDS had been distorted and the facts exaggerated.

'We really wanted you to come on to the programme and talk about some of the problems likely to be caused by the disease,' persisted the researcher.

'I'm happy to come on to the programme and say that I think that the dangers posed by the disease have been exaggerated,' I told the researcher.

The researcher sighed. 'Quite a few doctors have said that to me,' he said sadly. 'But it really isn't the sort of angle we're looking for.'

Very gently I put down the telephone. I didn't expect to hear from the researcher again and I didn't. His company produced a television programme about AIDS that appeared on our screens a short time after that conversation. And I suspect that most of those who viewed it went to bed believing that AIDS was the greatest threat to mankind since the Black Death.

That was by no means an isolated incident. The facts about AIDS were carefully selected to satisfy the public image of the disease — and to satisfy those with vested interests to protect.

15

At the time when that television company was broadcasting a programme predicting that AIDS would soon affect us all the official figures showed that just eight heterosexuals had contracted AIDS in Britain. That wasn't the total for one year. It was the total for ever.

To try to put this in perspective I wrote an article at the time pointing out that in Britain during the previous two years no less than thirty six people had died while horse riding.

16

According to experts speaking in the late 1980s on behalf of the Government and the British Medical Association, AIDS was likely to decimate the British population before the decade was out. (There were at the time considerably more so-called experts on AIDS than there were patients with AIDS).

Politicians and the medical experts agreed that within a few years every family in the country would be affected by the disease. An official spokesman for the British Medical Association (the doctors' trade union) was widely quoted as forecasting that within five years 400 people a month would be dying of the disease, though as far as I know no one bothered to ask him where he got this figure from. It was officially forecast that every family in the UK would soon be touched by AIDS and one gloomy official forecast was that by the year 2000 we would all have the disease. The Government paid a fortune to put bizarre advertisements involving icebergs on television screens. These, it was rumoured, had something to do with AIDS and were intended as a warning to us all.

17

Back in 1988 I pointed out that two specific groups had been particularly at risk: syringe sharing drug users and promiscuous homosexuals.

'These two groups are at risk because AIDS is essentially a disease that is transmitted through the blood (rather than a sexually transmitted disease) and both these groups enjoy practices which involve possible contamination through an exchange of blood.'

One of the most significant scientific papers available then concluded that the only sexual practice which was found likely to lead to contracting AIDS was receptive anal intercourse. Another important study showed that on average homosexuals who contracted AIDS had had 1,100 sexual partners.

This evidence was available in medical and scientific journals. But AIDS had become so fashionable that no one was interested in anything as boring as evidence.

18

Why was the threat of AIDS exaggerated so recklessly?

In my book *The Health Scandal* I put forward a number of possible explanations.

First, I explained that AIDS was an attractive media disease. People love being terrified. Aware of this television companies are constantly on the look out for new scare stories. That television researcher I spoke to wasn't the only person working in television who wanted to build up the myth about AIDS.

A killer disease that is transmitted sexually made irresistible copy. For example, it enabled the religious right to tell those whom they regarded as promiscuous that AIDS was a sign of the wrath of God. Television producers could confront people who believed in free love with people who disapproved of any sex outside marriage. And, best of all, producers could make programmes in which eager experts showed viewers how a condom should be put onto a penis.

Second, AIDS had by 1988 become big business. And it was making a lot of money for a lot of people. Medical researchers admitted to me that they found it much easier to get funding for projects if their project title had the disease AIDS mentioned in it. Private screening clinics were making a fortune. Companies making drugs which were recommended for patients thought to have AIDS found that their share prices rocketed. Shares in the drug company which had produced an anti-AIDS drug called AZT, rocketed by 360% in just twelve months. A portfolio of shares in companies offering AIDS solutions rose by a magnificent 41%.

19

When I was eventually allowed into radio studios to discuss AIDS I took part in a radio programme with a spokesman for a group of homosexuals who had been loudly promoting the theory that AIDS was a heterosexual disease. On the programme I read from scientific papers which proved conclusively that the risks to heterosexuals were extremely slight. But the spokesman for the homosexuals ignored my evidence, and without any of his own, insisted that AIDS was a threat to us all. After the programme we stood together on the pavement outside the studio waiting for taxis. I asked him why he persisted with an argument which he must have known was not based on science. Away from the microphone he was honest. 'If we admit that AIDS is a disease which affects gays no one will be interested in it and no one will do any research into it,' he admitted.

And that was the truth. Gay pressure groups (working to make sure that AIDS did not become established as a 'gay' disease') were responsible for the initial development of the 'plague' myth. AIDS was then turned into a major scare through the efforts of insurance companies (eager to find an excuse to put up premiums), drug companies (keen to sell new products), doctors (keen to help drug companies), researchers (eager to get their hands on the vast amounts of money being raised by volunteers), religious groups (desperate to exploit an opportunity to suppress sexual activity outside marriage) and politicians (eager, as always, to leap on an opportunity to frighten the voters — since when voters are frightened it is much easier to introduce new, repressive legislation).

20

During the late 1980s the mail I received from readers of my newspaper and magazine columns proved to me that the AIDS propaganda campaigns had affected the lives of millions of men and women who had absolutely no risk at all of contracting the disease. So, for example, I received a sad letter from a 57-year-old widow who had been to her doctor for an internal examination. She was worried that if the doctor had previously examined a patient with AIDS she might have caught the disease. She told me that she wouldn't be going back to the doctor unless I could provide her with reassurance. Another letter came from a reader who wanted to know if her small son could have caught AIDS from an insect bite. There were letters from an old lady who wouldn't pat her dog in case she caught AIDS from it and a worried mother whose son wouldn't kiss her goodnight for fear of catching AIDS. And Michael Coles was by no means the only person to kill himself as a result of all the AIDS scaremongering.

In 1988, I wrote that I strongly suspected that the scare campaign about AIDS had killed more heterosexuals than the disease itself. I am now convinced that I was absolutely right.

21

Telling the truth about AIDS was not easy. Indeed, for most of the time, it was very nearly impossible. When a disease becomes fashionable, and is promoted by the whole of the establishment, anyone who stands against the storm of support must expect to be under pressure.

When my book *The Health Scandal* was being prepared for publication in 1988 the publishers (Sidgwick and Jackson) were wildly enthusiastic about its prospects and expressed themselves eager to promote the book as widely as possible.

But suddenly, and without explanation, things changed. The book came out without even a whimper — let alone a bang. There was so little publicity that I sent out a press release myself — and was actually told off by the publishers for doing so. The book was remaindered very quickly and no real effort was made to sell the paperback rights. (Indeed, Sidgwick and Jackson insisted that the paperback rights could not be sold because no one wanted to buy them. My agent took back the rights and sold the paperback rights very quickly. This was curious because it meant that we did not have to share the financial proceeds from the paperback sale with Sidgwick and Jackson). I got the impression that a book of mine had been effectively suppressed by its own publisher.

22

When, in 1989, I talked about my book *Sex For Everyone* to the publisher's representatives, publicity department and editorial staff many of the audience started to walk out when I claimed that AIDS was not a major threat to heterosexuals. (The publisher was called Angus and Robertson but the audience also included many employees of associated companies.)

The trickle of people leaving the room turned into a flood when I suggested that the campaign to prevent AIDS should adopt the phrase 'Stop buggering about' as a slogan. The ignorance of these people (many of whom seemed to regard themselves as knowledgeable but who were instead sanctimonious and egregiously ill-informed) was typical at the time. After my speech had finished a number of stunningly ignorant people came up to me and told me that they would not help promote or sell the book because they regarded my claims that AIDS was not a serious threat to heterosexuals as grossly irresponsible. Indignant and self-righteous editorial employees glowered at me and did their best to make me feel unwelcome. I remember feeling so unwelcome that I left the hotel very late at night and drove several hundred miles back home in the dark rather than use the bedroom that had been reserved for me.

The book's sales were duly disastrous, destroyed by its publisher because I had dared to tell the truth and expose the AIDS myth for what it was.

23

When I first criticised the highly fashionable AIDS myth I was vilified for daring even to suggest that AIDS might not be the heterosexual epidemic the Government, the medical establishment and the media was warning us about.

According to former *Sunday Times* Editor Andrew Neil, the same thing happened to American author Michael Fumento who wrote a book called *The Myth of Heterosexual Aids.*

Neil recalls that; 'Instead of confronting Fumento's arguments and figures, the Aids Lobby resorted to abusing him for daring to write such a book...I began to think that maybe all this bluster was to hide the truth: there was no heterosexual epidemic.'

24

I remember going to a medical bookshop in the early 1990s and being appalled to see shelf after shelf of books about AIDS and very few books at all about cancer. At the time anyone with AIDS would end up surrounded by would-be helpers. Anyone with cancer would have to wait months, even years, for treatment

25

The scientific evidence and the figures available when the AIDS fashion was at its greatest, proved conclusively that there was no AIDS epidemic among heterosexuals and that there never would be. Since the 1980s and early 1990s the evidence has continued to support this viewpoint.

The AIDS myth was deliberately created by homosexuals who feared, probably correctly, that if AIDS was thought to be a disease which only affected homosexuals it would not receive much funding. The myth was sustained by a variety of self-serving groups.

The billions of pounds that have been pumped into the AIDS industry have resulted in the development of a massive industry of helpers, advisors, aides and so on.

Most of those involved in raising, distributing and spending this money knew and know little or nothing about the disease and although some were probably well-intentioned there were far more of them than there were alleged AIDS sufferers.

The AIDS fashionistas have continued to defend their industry with great enthusiasm and commitment, largely because it is their jobs and their industry they are defending.

26

There is still much mystery about whether the HIV virus really exists and, if it does exist, whether it has anything to do with AIDS.

Just one thing is crystal clear: the predictions of the medical establishment, the politicians and the journalists who claimed that by the end of the 20th century one in three of us would be touched by AIDS were absurd scaremongering.

27

Claims that Africa is ravaged by AIDS are also misleading and dangerous. If there is AIDS in Africa then it is because anal sex is widespread in African countries (where it is used as a form of birth control) and because a scarcity of doctors and treatments means that venereal diseases (creating bleeding sores) are widespread too.

In order to justify the huge expenditure of time and money on research into finding a cure many of those involved in helping to maintain the AIDS industry have for years been busily changing the rules about the way that AIDS is defined.

These days if you die of influenza, malaria or tuberculosis (TB) in Africa there is a good chance that you will be included in the AIDS statistics.

(Including TB and malaria victims in the AIDS statistics is one of the ways in which the alleged AIDS plague in Africa has been created. This type of 'bending' of the statistics is nothing new. When the authorities wanted to give the impression that smallpox had been conquered by the vaccination programme they attributed many deaths caused by smallpox to chickenpox — even though chickenpox is very rarely a fatal disease.)

Describing diseases such as tuberculosis and malaria, which are well-established in Africa, and which are a real threat, as AIDS is tragic. The end result is that more money is handed to AIDS researchers and AIDS agencies and less is given to controlling real and well-established killer diseases such as tuberculosis and malaria. It is hardly surprising that the death rate from AIDS is said to be exploding. People aren't really dying of AIDS; they are dying of tuberculosis and malaria.

28

I have no doubt that the enormously fashionable AIDS industry, in its various discredited forms, has now killed far more people than the disease. But perhaps the most worrying thing about AIDS is that the truth about the disease is never acknowledged or discussed by AIDS experts, by people working in the AIDS industry or by the mainstream media.

AIDS has become a sacred disease.

To question the motives of those involved in the search for a vaccine or a cure, or the treatment of alleged AIDS patients, is politically incorrect and utterly unacceptable.

And, of course, those members of the media who leapt on the AIDS bandwagon in the 1980s and early 1990s are probably too embarrassed to want to talk about their mistakes.

29

The AIDS story is a good example of the way that doctors cause more fear than they ease. (They create the fear to suit the needs of governments and corporations.)

Experts always exaggerate the importance of their subject in order to make themselves appear more important than they are.

For example, just as the people who warn constantly about AIDS are looking for fame and money so many of the people who warn about bird 'flu are all bird 'flu experts with, inevitably, both a vested interest in creating interest in their speciality and in some cases a commercial interest in selling remedies.

30

Psychiatrists and psychologists are eager to create fashionable new bandwagons too. It is now possible to be clinically afraid of 530 different things, for that is the astonishing number of phobias which have been officially recognised. In addition to traditional phobias such as claustrophobia patients can now suffer from kakorrhaphiophobia (a fear of defeat), apeirophobia (a fear of infinity), chrometophobia (a fear of money) and hippopotomonstros-esquippedaliphobia (a fear of long words). It's difficult to tell when they're being serious and when they're having us on these days. (But these *are* real.)

31

Drug companies exaggerate mild problems in order to boost their profits and they devise and then promote non-existent diseases in order to create new markets for their drugs.

In our book *How To Conquer Health Problems Between Ages 50 and 120* my wife (Donna Antoinette Coleman) and I described how drug companies had marketed hormone replacement therapy for so-called menopausal problems (and done so with such vigour and skill that one third of postmenopausal women use hormone replacement therapy and are, presumably, unaware that it may increase the risk of developing breast cancer, heart disease, stroke and gall bladder attack) and how they had built up osteoporosis as a disease requiring long-term, expensive preventive therapy when in fact it requires nothing of the sort.

32

Many so-called disease awareness campaigns are in practice drug company marketing programmes, designed not to educate people how to avoid ill health but, rather, to persuade them to take drugs. Doctors, nurses and people who think they are campaigning on behalf of patients (and whose motives may be honourable) are, too often, manipulated into helping to fulfil the commercial ambitions of ruthless drug companies.

33

One of the most absurd of the new and most fashionable diseases is 'chronic obstructive pulmonary disease'.

According to drug company sponsored experts, COPD now affects three million people in the UK alone (with two thirds of them Still undiagnosed, untreated and, therefore, a huge reservoir of potential profit).

COPD didn't exist at all in Britain a few years ago and the drug companies and experts who imported this new disease from the USA (where it has become enormously successful and has for some years been one of the biggest profit spinners for the pharmaceutical industry) claim that it usually affects smokers over the age of 35 and it often involves a cough and daytime breathlessness.

Curiously enough those are the very same symptoms which used to be ascribed to a disease known as emphysema. Emphysema was never very profitable because doctors recognised that there wasn't a great deal they could do for it. Saying that someone is breathless because they smoke isn't much of a disease and there isn't, therefore, much chance to provide profitable treatment. How can drug companies (or doctors) make big profits out of telling people to give up smoking?

Patients who suffered from emphysema and chronic bronchitis (though different, the two diseases were usually related and patients often had both) were good customers for antibiotic therapy but that was about all. They weren't of much interest to drug companies searching for new ways to make bigger profits.

And so some bright spark imported COPD: a wonderful sounding disease for which a whole host of powerful and expensive drug therapies (including anti-'flu vaccinations, steroid inhalers, antibiotics, tranquillisers, sleeping tablets and anti-depressants) are now recommended. Most of the big drug companies have leapt upon this bandwagon. In the UK the 'market opportunity' is said to be expected to grow to £6 billion by the year 2010. Naturally, these powerful and expensive drug therapies produce dozens of side effects which require numerous additional prescriptions. COPD is a drug industry dream; a chronic cash bonanza. Maybe they should have been honest and called the disease Chronic Drug Company Profit Maker and given it the acronym CDCPM.

34

In the UK, to encourage general practitioners to diagnose plenty of patients as COPD sufferers, family doctors who manage to make enough diagnoses will receive an annual cash bonus.

35

Some of the most important contributions made by doctors to the health of their patients have involved the cessation of harmful but fashionable practices.

So, for example, when doctors stopped bleeding their patients a century ago they saved many lives.

Just under a century ago bromides were recognised as dangerous and used accordingly by the more thoughtful prescribers. Barbiturates were widely recommended as the safe alternative. Then, half a century ago barbiturates were found to be dangerous. Amphetamines were recommended as safe. Then they were found to be addictive. Benzodiazepines were recommended as safe alternatives for barbiturates. Then they too were found to be too dangerous for general long-term use.

On each occasion that a group of drugs was found to be dangerous some doctors made their names by taking their patients off those drugs. So, for example, at least one doctor became famous after taking patients off bromides. Liberated from their drug-induced stupor his patients cheered him loudly.

Sadly, in many cases, these doctors then made the mistake of starting their patients on the newer and more fashionable product.

36

Surgeons, like physicians and general practitioners, have always been dedicated followers of fashion.

Back in the 19th century one of the most fashionable operations was the removal of lengths of intestine from patients complaining of constipation. A surgeon called Arbuthnot Lane achieved great fame and accumulated enormous wealth as a result of removing a cumulative total of several miles of intestine from his patients. Sadly, the patients didn't do as well without their intestines as Arbuthnot did with their money. The patients developed diarrhoea and lived miserable lives.

An American doctor, Dr Harry C. Sharp of the Jeffersonville Reformatory in Indiana, USA, performed 176 vasectomies on boys who had admitted to having masturbated. He claimed that his sterilised young patients slept better, felt better and had better appetites and he insisted that the operation made them stronger in mind and body. For reasons I cannot begin to imagine, Sharp also performed 280 vasectomies on patients suffering from colour blindness or defective vision.

In the 1930's, destructive brain surgery became fashionable after American workers removed the frontal lobes of chimpanzees and reported that the animals seemed more contented afterwards. In 1936 a neurosurgeon working in Portugal decided to test the theory by performing a variation of the operation on humans. He injected alcohol into the frontal lobes of 20 schizophrenics. After he claimed success for his operation other surgeons developed other techniques for destroying parts of the brain. An American surgeon called Walter Freeman of Washington University performed thousands of operations in which he simply cut off the frontal lobes of his patients. As long ago as 1971 it was estimated that this enormously fashionable operation (leucotomy) had been performed on over 100,000 patients. It was recommended as a treatment for patients who had been diagnosed as suffering from schizophrenia, depression, obsessional neurosis, anxiety state, hysteria, eczema, asthma, chronic rheumatism, anorexia nervosa, ulcerative colitis, tuberculosis, hypertension, angina, pain and anxiety caused by barbiturate toxicity.

Surgeons admitted that 'the more subtle powers of the intellect, such as its intuitive and imaginative qualities, may sometimes be affected detrimentally' but regarded this as a small price to pay. Complications of the operation also included bed-wetting, somnolence, severe and prolonged confusion and paralysis. Some patients developed epilepsy after the operation. Others had damaged personalities. All the patients I've met who have had this operation have behaved more like zombies than like human beings.

Although this operation is nowhere near as fashionable as it used to be, it's still being performed. As is electroconvulsive therapy (ECT) which I described in my book *How To Stop Your Doctor Killing You.*

Today, there are a number of fashionable operations. Surgeons are removing pieces of stomach or intestine from overweight patients (so that they will digest less of their food and, therefore, lose weight). These operations have been popular for several decades but are still remarkably fashionable. The side effects are horrendous and can include the metabolic problems inevitably produced by the diarrhoea and malabsorption and malnutrition which result from the fact that the body does not absorb the nutrients it needs. The excessive diarrhoea associated with some operations can result in potassium, magnesium and calcium depletion. Patients also stand a good chance of developing kidney stones and nearly half develop pains similar to rheumatoid arthritis in their joints. There is, of course, also the not inconsiderable risk that the patient will die on the operating table. The normal risks of anaesthesia are increased when the patient is overweight as, by definition, patients having this operation will be.

The removal of healthy breasts from young women has in recent years developed into a small epidemic. The breasts are removed so that they cannot become cancerous and the surgeons recommending the operation claim that it helps protect women who have a genetic susceptibility to breast cancer. I wonder how many of the women who are subjected to this mutilation are advised that their chances of developing breast cancer may also be reduced by eating a low fat vegetarian diet. Still, an operation is easier isn't it?

One surgeon who advocates breast removal as a way of avoiding breast cancer claims that 57% of women are at high risk of developing breast cancer and that these women should all have prophylactic (preventive) bilateral mastectomies and have their breast tissue replaced with silicone implants.

Other advocates of breast removal are less dramatic and claim that the operation need only be performed on a smaller group of women.

But is there any evidence to support the idea that removing breasts is a wise way to avoid cancer?

I don't think so. Even among women who carry the BRCA1 and BRCA2 breast cancer genes, and who have a strong family history of breast cancer, there are many other factors to take into consideration. Most women who are regarded as 'high risk' for breast cancer don't die of breast cancer, even if they keep both their breasts. Some die of breast cancer even after both healthy breasts have been removed. Some will undoubtedly die of complications as a result of the prophylactic surgery. I suspect that for many of the women who are subjected to the removal of healthy breasts the operation leads to a loss of quality of life without any prolongation of life.

Saddest of all is the fact that I have never heard any advocate of this type of operation point out to potential 'patients' that their susceptibility to breast cancer is just that: an extra susceptibility. A woman who has a family history of breast cancer may be more likely to develop breast cancer but she won't necessarily get it. And any woman who is susceptible to breast cancer can dramatically reduce her chances of developing the disease by avoiding the factors known to increase her risk.

Would women who are genetically susceptible to breast cancer dramatically improve their chances of avoiding the disease if they cut down their intake of fatty food, avoided meat and lost any excess weight?

The evidence suggests that they would.

Would such women be better protected than if they had their breasts removed?

I suspect that they would.

But as far as I have been able to find out no one has yet done any research to find out.

37

Removing teeth used to be extremely fashionable. The most enthusiastic dentist of all time was probably Brother Giovanni Battista Orsenigo who practised in Rome at the end of the 19th century. Brother Orsenigo kept all the teeth he pulled and in 1903 they were counted. It turned out that he had removed over two million teeth in his career — that works out at an average of 185 teeth a day. Not many modern dentists could equal that workload.

38

A reader of mine who had had a cancerous growth wrote to me. 'The cancer was removed by a surgeon who told me that the cancer had not spread,' she wrote. 'But doctors want me to have radiotherapy. Why?'

The answer is simple and shocking.

Radiotherapists want to prove that radiotherapy works. (There is at present surprisingly little evidence for its effectiveness.)

The current way to measure the effectiveness of treatments is to see how many patients survive for five years after diagnosis.

By giving treatment to patients who may not really need it — and who are likely to make a full recovery whether or not they receive treatment — doctors can make their pet therapy look good. But radiotherapy, which is currently very fashionable, can be extremely dangerous. It may (or may not) kill more people than it saves. No one really knows.

Amazingly there are no firm rules about who must get radiotherapy — or how much they should receive.

Local doctors decide how much radiotherapy to give and for how long. Orthodox cancer therapy is, I'm afraid, just as wishy washy and disorganised as alternative cancer therapy. And it's far more dangerous. Radiotherapy can seriously damage your health.

This is a scandal of monumental proportions.

So, how do doctors decide who gets radiotherapy and how much they get?'

If you don't want to know look away now.

Because the answer may frighten you.

They guess.

Radiotherapy is a lottery and (like chemotherapy) about as logical as drinking your own urine or standing in the garden chanting to the moon.

I invited the British Government to comment on this scandal.

Their first attempt was:

'We work in close consultation with royal (sic) colleges and professional societies who produce detailed guidance on cancer therapy, including chemotherapy and radiotherapy. The Department of Health provides broad information on the use of chemotherapy and radiotherapy which acts as guidance for trained consultants.'

This is, of course, meaningless drivel of the sort for which governments and bureaucrats everywhere are famous.

So I rang up and tried to make things simple. 'Does a woman in Cornwall who has breast cancer get the same radiotherapy treatment as a woman in Leeds who has the same type of breast cancer.'

That seemed straightforward enough.

Here is the Department of Health's second attempt:

'Guidelines are established so that patients receive care from a multidisciplinary team, the same treatments are available to patients, and professional advice is available for consultants to ensure patients receive appropriate treatment for their condition.'

Leaving aside the barefaced lie ('the same treatments are available to patients') and removing the lexicological debris we are left with: 'professional advice is available for consultants to ensure patients receive appropriate treatment'.

And that is fine and dandy if consultants ask for advice. What the Department of Health clearly does not do is provide consultant radiotherapists (or physicians prescribing chemotherapy) with any firm guidelines about how much therapy, how often and for how long.

So how do consultants decide what therapy to give their patients?

They guess.

We should not, I suppose, be too surprised.

For that, after all, is what doctors do every time they reach for a prescription pad.

Don't ever let any doctor tell you that alternative medicine is unscientific.

39

The medical profession and the media seem to vie with one another in creating fashionable new diseases out of problems and fears which people have lived with for centuries. Unhappiness or disappointments are labelled as depression (and treated with drugs). A single bout of wheezing is dignified as asthma and requires life-long treatment with powerful drugs which, as I have been pointing out for decades, can kill. A patch of dry skin becomes eczema and requires treatment with heavy-duty steroid creams. Baldness, once just something that happened to men with the passing of time, is now widely regarded as an illness which needs to be treated with powerful drugs or extravagant surgery. Obesity isn't a consequence of over-eating but a sign of glandular dysfunction requiring therapeutic intervention. Women who have smaller than average breasts are described as 'suffering' from a disease labelled as 'micromastia'. Shyness has been relabelled 'social anxiety syndrome'. And on it goes, and will doubtless continue to go.

When I first introduced the concept of stress as a cause of disease in a book called *Stress Control* (in the 1970s) I was reviled and sneered at by doctors and journalists. One Medical School Professor announced that I should be struck off the medical register for suggesting that there might be a link between stress and disease. Today stress (a serious cause of ill health) is now so fashionable and devalued as a concept that one in four people is said to be suffering from mental illness caused by stress.

Women who carry heavy shopping bags are officially categorised as 'disabled' (whether or not they have any difficulty in carrying their bags). In America there are 30 million women suffering from 'hurried women syndrome' and 43% of women are allegedly suffering from something called 'female sexual dysfunction'.

And people who work at nights are said to suffer from 'chronic shift work sleep disorder' rather than just having difficulty sleeping in the daytime.

40

Finally, one of the most fashionable medical interventions today is undoubtedly vaccination. A generation or two ago children obtained immunity to childhood diseases (chicken pox, measles and mumps) by attending parties. All the children in the neighbourhood would be invited round for tea and games if a child contracted one of the common (but relatively unthreatening) childhood diseases. Those children attending the party who contracted the disease would put up with spots for a week or so and then recover. Parents would, probably justifiably, assume that a child who hadn't caught the disease had probably acquired immunity to it. The system was simple, uneventful and relatively safe.

These days children have vaccinations. Loads of them. It is the fashion. It is our way. Drug companies and doctors make huge amounts of money out of it.

Coleman's 8ᵗʰ Law Of Medicine

The medical establishment will always take decisions on health matters which benefit industry, government and the medical profession, rather than patients. And the government will always take decisions on health matters which benefit the State rather than individual patients. What you read, hear or see about medicine and health matters will have more to do with the requirements of the pharmaceutical industry and the government, than the genuine needs of patients.

1

Around the world populations are ruled by nonentities blessed only with enough ambition and greed to get into power, enough dishonesty to disguise their incompetence and sufficient ruthlessness and lack of imagination to ensure that they never feel shame or embarrassment. These so-called leaders will cling to power whatever may happen. This is as true of the medical establishment as it is of governments.

2

Responsibility has been separated from authority with disastrous consequences for patients. Your chances of getting the best treatment for your condition depend not upon your needs but upon a whole range of factors such as political correctness, expediency and (as I explained in Coleman's 7th Law Of Medicine) fashion. While people with suspected cancer have to wait months for essential investigations our politically correct system means that money and resources are spent on providing such non-essential luxuries as cosmetic surgery and infertility treatment It is society's choice to spend its limited resources in this way (largely because of pressure from loud-mouthed campaigners representing specific points of view). There is something uncivilised and inhuman about a health system in which patients with suspected cancer must wait and wait to be diagnosed and then wait and wait to be treated — hoping that they won't die on one of the waiting lists — while patients requiring cosmetic surgery or treatment for infertility get treated ahead of them. In any State run health service financial resources must be finite: not everyone can get everything they want. But the way patients are chosen for treatment is appallingly cruel and quite indefensible.

3

The failure of governments and doctors to ensure that health care services are fair and reasonable may affect your life in a very dramatic way. You should, therefore, be prepared with alternatives. For example, you should have enough money in the bank to enable you to pay for crucial investigations should they be necessary. Once you have been diagnosed as suffering from a life-threatening condition doctors, nurses and administrators may find it harder to deny you essential treatment.

4

Our governments and doctors have allowed our environment and our food to be poisoned by chemical companies, farmers and others involved in 'serving' our communities.

Poisons in our environment are now one of the most significant modern causes of illness in general and of cancer in particular. As a result of the contaminants in our food, drinking water and the air we breathe, human breast milk contains so many chemical contaminants that it couldn't possibly be sold as safe for human consumption. And human bodies contain so many chemicals (some consumed in additive and pesticide contaminated food and some acquired accidentally from our polluted environment) that a human steak would never be passed fit for consumption by cannibals.

Children's bodies are routinely contaminated with scores of potentially hazardous chemicals. The susceptibility of the young body, and the wide availability of toxic chemicals in the surroundings in which children live, mean that those as young as nine years old have far more toxic substances in their bodies than their grandparents ever had.

Television sets and plastic toys, deodorants and household cleansers are all sources of poisons as, of course, are the pesticides we use in our garden and the pesticides farmers use on our food.

Some carcinogenic industrial chemicals which have been banned can still be found in the environment. Back in 1930 just one million tons of man-made chemicals were produced globally each year. Today, the chemical companies produce 400 million tons of man-made chemicals a year.

When researchers tested ordinary citizens they found that of 104 substances for which they had tested, 80 were present in human beings. There was little correlation between where people live and the chemicals they have in their bodies. Living in the country is no protection. Chemicals are in our air, our water and our food. The chemicals found in the average human body can cause liver cancer, damage to the developing brain, premature birth, genital abnormalities, bladder cancer, kidney damage, asthma, skin disorders, hormone disruption, and a higher risk of miscarriage.

5

Tests done in the early 21st century showed that the blood of health and environment ministers from 13 European Union (EU) countries was contaminated with dozens of industrial chemicals — including some that were banned decades ago.

The tests, conducted on EU ministers from Great Britain, Cyprus, the Czech Republic, Denmark, Estonia, France, Finland, Hungary, Italy, Lithuania, Slovakia, Sweden and Spain showed that the politicians had an average of 37 industrial chemicals in their blood. The ministers were found to have a total of 55 different industrial chemicals in their blood. One minister had 45 chemicals in his blood. The 'cleanest' had 33.

The chemicals included those used in fire-resistant furniture, non-stick pans, greaseproof boxes, fragrances and pesticides. Unsurprisingly, the effects and dangers of the chemicals involved were, it was admitted largely unknown.

6

There is not enough safety information available about nearly 90% of the 2,500 chemicals which manufacturers regularly use in large quantities to enable scientists or doctors to do a basic safety assessment.

The tests done on EU ministers were used to support an EU proposal known as REACH (Registration, Evaluation and Authorisation of Chemicals) in which thousands of chemicals will be tested on millions of animals. If the tests show that a chemical doesn't hurt animals the substance will be given a clean bill of health and manufacturers will be allowed to use it as much as they like. If the tests show that a chemical kills animals the test will be ignored on the grounds that animals are so different to humans that the results are irrelevant and manufacturers will be allowed to use the chemical as much as they like.

You think I'm joking don't you? Or being unduly cynical? I'm not. I'm being deadly serious.

The EU is deliberately designing and performing safety tests to be performed on animals. These, they know, will prove nothing but the tests will satisfy those who are concerned about carcinogenic chemicals without harming the profitability of the industries involved.

Incidentally, exactly the same flawed and pointless tests are being duplicated in the United States of America.

7

There is no doubt at all that many of the chemicals widely used in the preparation of food, the feeding of animals and the manufacture of a wide variety of goods are carcinogenic — they cause cancer.

But what do doctors do about all this?

Nothing.

Absolutely nothing.

8

Since 19821 have been arguing that the drinking water from our taps is now unsafe to drink because it contains pharmaceutical residues. People who drink tap water are drinking second hand drug residues. (There is more on this in my books *Food for Thought, How To Stop Your Doctor Killing You* and *Superbody*.)

The basic problem is that after a drug is swallowed much of the compound is excreted in urine and will end up contaminating drinking water. So when you turn on your tap you get bits of old contraceptive pill, antibiotic and tranquilliser in your nice sparkling glass of apparently clean drinking water. You can't see the drug residues, of course. And the water companies can't get them out.

From time to time newspapers and magazines around the world discover some new research showing that male fish are changing sex in drug polluted rivers (it is, of course, the female hormones from contraceptive pills and hormone replacement therapy which cause this particular problem) but once they realise the size of the problem they soon back off and forget about the story.

9

Governments have, of course, made things worse by adding fluoride to drinking water supplies. The theory is that if people drink water dosed with fluoride they will be less likely to suffer from dental decay. In practice, fluoride is a potentially dangerous substance and this practice is fraught with danger. Adding fluoride to the water is, however, encouraged by politicians because although it probably damages the health of some citizens it may help cut the nation's dental bill.

10

Some countries now force the manufacturers of flour to add folic acid to their product. This is done in both the USA and Canada, and other governments seem keen to follow suit. The clinical argument for contaminating food in this way is that adding folic acid to flour and bread will help prevent relatively rare (but expensive to treat) conditions such as spina bifida and other neural tube defects in newborn babies. The financial argument in favour is that this will save the country money (and, presumably, help increase profits for the manufacturers of folic acid). The arguments against forcibly adding folic acid to flour and bread are that women who are planning to get pregnant can take folic add supplements if they wish (or can simply increase their intake of foods rich in the vitamin) without the rest of the population being forcibly medicated. More seriously, there is some evidence suggesting that folic add might increase the risk of bowel cancer developing and the presence of folic add in bread will undoubtedly make it difficult for doctors to diagnose vitamin B12 deficiency in patients. Vitamin B12 deficiency can lead to neurological problems such as memory loss and a lack of limb control but it is most commonly found in the elderly and so few politicians or campaigners are bothered about this.

The big question, of course, is where will this lead? If campaigners and drug companies succeed in convincing politicians that it is in their interest to put folic add in a basic foodstuff how much longer will it be before someone convinces politicians that they will benefit if tranquillisers are put into chocolate, baked beans or drinking water?

11

Don't buy purified water. Buy pure, natural, mineral spring water.

Coca Cola withdrew its Dasani brand of bottled water after the product was found to contain illegal levels of a potentially harmful chemical. Dasani wasn't a natural spring water but was simply tap water which had allegedly been purified to remove all the bacteria and minerals. The problem was that the 'purified' water contained excess levels of bromate, a chemical which can increase the risk of cancer if you are exposed to it for a long time. (And drinking water is, for most people, a pretty long-term activity).

Coca Cola said that the elevated levels of bromate came as a result of the calcium chloride they had added to the water to meet a UK legal requirement.

12

When the American Environmental Protection Agency tested the water provided by passenger airlines they found that on many occasions the planes were carrying drinking water which failed tests because it contained coliform bacteria such as e.coli. An air transport association spokesmen said that the airlines were confident that their drinking water was safe. But then they would, wouldn't they?

13

As part of a school science project a 12-year-old American girl collected ice samples from five restaurants in South Florida. She also collected toilet water samples from the same restaurants. She had all the samples tested for bacteria at the University of South Florida.

In several cases the ice from the restaurants contained e.coli bacteria and was dirtier than the water taken from the toilet bowls. How did the bugs get into the ice?

Probably because the ice making machines hadn't been cleaned and because the restaurant staff had use hands which hadn't been washed to scoop up the ice.

The moral is a simple one: you should avoid ice in bars and restaurants.

The first question is: why did it take a 12-year-old girl to expose this sort of contamination?

The second question is: has anything been done about it?

(That's a rhetorical question to which both you and I know the answer.)

14

Taxes are used to create huge bureaucracies. Once the bureaucracy has been developed money has to be raised to sustain the bureaucracy, which becomes more important than anything else. If there is a shortage of money in hospitals doctors and nurses are fired — not administrators.

15

You shouldn't eat food which has been imported from the USA.

America still allows its farmers to use the pesticide methyl bromide, even though the chemical has been banned elsewhere under the 1987 Montreal Protocol because of its contribution to the global warming problem. Methyl bromide is widely used by American tomato and strawberry farmers but has been linked to prostate cancer and to neurological damage. The Bush administration obtained an exemption for the poison on the grounds that it is popular among farmers.

Methyl bromide is also used to fumigate food processing and storage areas, such as grain bins and flour mills, where it is used to kill insects and rats.

16

Meat and milk from cloned animals will be on sale soon. An American Government report, from the Food and Drug Administration, has concluded that 'cloned animal products appear to be safe for consumption'. Consumers should be terrified by the carefree way with which the American Government includes, but ignores, the word 'appear'. The long-term effects of eating cloned meat and milk are, of course, unknown.

17

The main reason for America's refusal to stick to its promise to ratify the Kyoto Treaty can be summed up in one word: money. American politicians put American business first, second and third. The world's people come nowhere. This philosophy is well illustrated by the way the Americans have dealt with Mad Cow Disease or BSE (bovine spongiform encephalopathy). Giving American cattle bone meal to eat was banned in 1997 but blood and gelatin were both made exempt from the ban. Only after confirming America's first case of mad cow disease did the American Government announce that cows which were too sick to walk would no longer be allowed into the food chain. Falling down — and not getting up again — is, of course, a well- known key symptom of mad cow disease and yet for years meat from hundreds of thousands of such animals — known as 'downers' had been packed up and sent to supermarkets.

18

An American dairy is being sued for claiming that the milk it sells contains no artificial growth hormones. It has been alleged that the dairy doesn't have the right to let its customers know whether or not its milk contains genetically engineered hormones. These hormones have been banned in just about every industrialised nation except America. The milk containing the hormones may cause cancer.

19

The Americans claim that giving hormones to cattle is perfectly safe. When hormone-rich beef from such cattle was banned in the EU the Americans responded by banning some European imports (more out of governmental spite than through any sense of commercial logic).

American farmers give six sex hormones to their cattle for exactly the same reason that bodybuilders and weight lifters take hormones: to build more muscle as quickly as possible. The benefit to a farmer is financial: there is obviously more saleable beef on a heavily muscled cow.

The row, which has been going on for well over a decade, is about whether or not beef taken from cows which have been given extra hormones is safe to eat. Although there is no evidence to show that hormone soaked beef is safe American farmers say that it is. And that, of course, is good enough for their Government. (All governments are as frightened of farmers as they are of any other big commercial lobby.)

However, European farmers are not allowed to give extra hormones to cattle. And so, not surprisingly, they have put pressure on European politicians to ban American beef (which, because of the help from the hormones, is cheaper to produce).

The American claim that it is safe to give hormones to cattle is based upon the fact that there is, as yet, not very much scientific proof that it is dangerous to do this.

This is exactly the same spurious argument that is used to defend genetic engineering, microwave ovens and other possible hazards to human health.

Everyone conveniently ignores the fact that it is extremely difficult to prove that something is dangerous when little or no research has been done to find the truth!

What we do know, however, is that the amount of hormone in a portion of meat can be more than a pubertal boy produces in a day. And that's a lot. And sex hormones can and do have a dramatic effect on any human body (and mind).

Moreover, research has been done showing that there is a convincing epidemiological link between one of the six hormones used by American farmers and endometrial and breast cancers. The hormone causes cancer by interfering with a cell's DNA — a process known as genotoxicity. It is generally accepted that there are no safe levels for genotoxic substances.

You might think that would be enough to embarrass the American politicians into telling their farmers to stop using hormones. After all, the incidence of cancer is rising dramatically in the USA — and has been doing so for some years. However, the American farmers (and their Government) have taken comfort from the fact that although a joint committee set up by the World Health Organisation and the Food and Agriculture Organisation has agreed that one of the hormones in use has what it calls 'genotoxic properties', and does cause cancer, it has argued that it is safe to allow people to consume modest amounts of this cancer-inducing hormone. Moreover, much to the delight of the Americans, the committee claims to know what the safe level is. You will not be surprised to hear that the American farmers and their Government claim that their beef contains less than this safe amount of this known cancer-inducing substance.

Anyone who eats American beef is playing a modern version of Russian roulette and is exhibiting an extraordinary amount of trust in a group of people (American politicians and American farmers) who have, in my view, consistently shown that they do not give a fig for human health or human life.

20

Fish farms supply almost all of the trout and catfish and half of the salmon and shrimp consumed in the USA.

Worldwide, one third of the seafood consumed is farmed fish.

However, a recent study showed that a single serving of farmed salmon contains three to six times the World Health Organisation's recommended daily intake limit for dioxins.

Farmed salmon (usually known as 'Atlantic salmon') are genetically modified to be larger (and therefore more profitable) than wild salmon. As a result a salmon farm which contains 200,000 fish releases nitrogen, phosphorus and faecal matter roughly equivalent to the untreated sewage from between 20,000 and 25,000 human beings.

One huge problem is that American fish farmers use a wide range of chemicals (including hormones, antibiotics, anaesthetics, pesticides etc.) in order to help increase their profits. The use of antibiotics by fish farmers is a particular hazard since it leads to antibiotic resistance.

21

Here's a simple example of the way commercial advantageous practices become accepted without there ever being any evidence to support them.

Cyclists are persuaded to wear helmets (if they are professional they are forced to wear them) although there doesn't seem to be any actual hard evidence that wearing helmets helps cyclists avoid serious injury. There are signs that governments will soon make it compulsory for all cyclists to wear helmets — whether they want to or not.

Research to prove that helmets did help would be easy enough to conduct (just find 1,000 cyclists who wear helmets and 1,000 who don't, making sure that they cycle in comparable circumstances, and at the end of a year find out how many in each group have had serious head injuries).

It is possible to argue that wearing helmets makes cycling more not less dangerous because they affect the weight of the head (and may, therefore, make an accident more likely or make a head injury more likely if you fall off). This is the sort of research Governments should do. No helmet manufacturer would do it (why should they?). But it is the sort of useful, practical, potentially life-saving research which is never, ever done. Instead a commercially useful myth becomes reality. Mobile phones are safe. Helmets for cyclists are essential.

22

There is something absurd, hypocritical and cruel about the way our governments bomb farmers who grow coca leaf and opium (both of which were relatively harmless substances until Western scientists refined them and turned them into more addictive drugs) while at the same time handing out huge subsidies to farmers growing tobacco (one of the world's most lethal products).

23

Breast cancer is an emotive subject which always gathers far more publicity than it might reasonably expect to receive. In Britain, the index to the Office of Health Economics Compendium of Health Statistics 2005-2006 contains five lines of references to breast cancer but no references at all for prostate cancer or bowel cancer.

Newspapers often suggest that breast cancer is the leading cause of death among women. It isn't. Heart disease is the leading cause of death among women. And lung cancer, not breast cancer, is, in most countries the cancer which kills most women. Judging by the photographs used to illustrate newspaper and magazine articles about breast cancer it is difficult to avoid the conclusion that the reason why the media concentrate on breast cancer to the exclusion of other diseases is that it gives them a politically correct excuse to publish photographs of semi-naked young women, though just why it is always considered necessary and proper to publish photos of naked breasts to illustrate an article about breast cancer is something of a mystery. No one, as far as I know, has ever illustrated an article about bowel cancer with a photograph of a length of bowel.

Most of the photographs of naked women are, of course, illustrations of pretty young women with firm, large breasts designed and destined to boost the publication's readership. This helps to boost the false impression that breast cancer is a disease which largely affects young women.

Sadly, women don't always benefit from the publicity given to breast cancer. Media campaigns often result in dangerously inappropriate testing being organised (such as widespread mammograms being made available for younger women) and in potentially dangerous and relatively untested drugs being promoted and sold.

24

The male disease which is directly comparable to breast cancer is, of course, prostate cancer. And yet prostate cancer (far more difficult to illustrate) only very rarely features in magazine and newspaper articles.

In the USA, for example, prostate cancer is far more frequent than breast cancer and kills approximately as many people. But whereas thousands of people run campaigns to find a cure for breast cancer very few run campaigns to find a cure for prostate cancer.

Prostate cancer is usually referred to in the media as an old person's disease. This simply isn't true. The figures for prostate cancer show that the incidence, age at diagnosis and mortality rates are very similar to those for breast cancer.

25

Colorectal cancer (cancers of the colon and rectum) is one of the commonest of all cancers and is a major killer of men and women. But not many people are encouraged by the media to walk around with ribbons pinned to their lapels showing that they are supporters of a campaign to stamp out colorectal cancer.

26

These days doctors only get to read and hear what the drug industry wants them to read and hear.

In July 2004 I was invited to speak at a conference in London. The conference was, I was told, intended to tackle the subject of medication errors and adverse reactions to prescribed drugs. The company organising the conference was called PasTest. 'For over thirty years PasTest has been providing medical education to professionals within the NHS,' they told me. 'Building on our commitment to quality in medical and healthcare education, PasTest is creating a range of healthcare events which focus on the professional development of clinicians and managers who are working together to deliver healthcare services for the UK. Our aim is to provide a means for those who are in a position to improve services on both national and regional levels. The topics covered by our conferences are embraced within policy, best practice, case study, clinical management and evidence based practice. PasTest endeavours to source the best speakers who will engage audiences with balanced, relevant and thought-provoking programmes. PasTest has proven in the past that by using thorough investigative research and keeping up-to-date with advances in healthcare and medical practice, a premium educational event can be achieved.'

Goody, I thought.

Iatrogenesis (doctor-induced disease) is something of a speciality of mine. I have written numerous books and articles on the subject. My campaigns have resulted in more drugs being banned or controlled than anyone else's.

In addition to my speaking at the conference the organisers wanted me to help them decide on the final programme. I thought the conference was an important one and would give me a good opportunity to tell NHS staff the truth. I signed a contract.

PasTest wrote to confirm my appointment as a consultant and speaker for the PasTest Conference Division. And then there was silence. My office repeatedly asked for details of when and where the conference was being held.

Silence.

Eventually a programme for the event appeared on the Internet. Curiously, my name was not on the list of speakers.

Here is part of the blurb promoting the conference:

'Against a background of increasing media coverage into the number of UK patients who are either becoming ill or dying due to adverse reactions to medication our conference aims to explain the current strategies to avoid Adverse Drug reactions and what can be done to educate patients.'

Putting the blame on patients for problems caused by prescription drugs is brilliant. Most drug related problems are caused by the stupidity of doctors not the ignorance of patients. If the aim is to educate patients on how best to avoid prescription drug problems the advice would be simple: 'Don't trust doctors.'

The promotion for the conference claims that 'It is estimated errors in medication...account for 4% of hospital bed capacity.' And that prescription drug problems 'reportedly kill up to 10,000 people a year in the UK'. As I would have shown (had I not been banned from the conference) these figures are absurdly low.

The list of speakers included a variety of people I had never heard of including one speaker representing The Association of the British Pharmaceutical Industry and another representing the Medicines and Healthcare Products Regulatory Agency.

Delegates representing the NHS were expected to pay £250 plus VAT (£293.75) to attend the event. Delegates whose Trust would be funding the cost were asked to apply for a Health Authority Approval form.

So why was I apparently banned from this conference?

This is what PasTest said when we asked them: 'certain parties felt that he (Vernon Coleman) was too controversial to speak and as a result would not attend.'

Could that, I wonder, be the drug industry? Is the drug industry now deciding whom they will allow to speak to doctors and NHS staff on the problems caused by prescription drugs? If I was banned at the behest of the drug industry do NHS bosses know that people attending such conferences will only hear speakers approved by the drug industry and that speakers telling the truth will be banned? (I think it is safe to assume that I won't be invited to speak at any more conferences for NHS staff.)

If I was banned at the behest of the medical profession why are doctors frightened of the truth? (If they think my views are wrong they would surely be happy for me to appear so that they could counter my arguments.)

I could not, of course, be banned by the NHS itself. Why would the NHS not want its employees to know the truth about drug-related problems?

Why are people who had me banned so frightened of what I would say? It can surely only be because they know that I would have caused embarrassment by telling the truth.

The scary bottom line is that the NHS paid a lot of money to send delegates to a conference where someone representing the drug industry spoke to them on drug safety. But I was banned. The truth was uninvited.

Because I had a contract, PasTest paid me *not* to turn up. I used the money to buy advertisements for my book *How To Stop Your Doctor Killing You.* Details of the ban were sent to every national and major local newspaper in Britain. None reported it.

27

Sadly, the truth is that doctors, administrators and drug companies all know that there are serious problems with the way health care is administered. But they would much rather sweep the problem under the carpet than have me lift the carpet, expose the full extent of the problem and threaten their cosy existence. Any system which cannot cope with real criticism is corrupt.

Doctors have to take back their traditional responsibility — and the authority (and power) that should always accompany responsibility.

28

You can no longer expect your conversations with your doctor to be treated as confidential.

Just two decades ago medical records were regarded as sacrosanct. Most doctors did everything they could to protect them from the eyes of social workers, policemen or other representatives of the State. Then, as the years went by, this level of confidentiality offered to patients began to diminish. The number of health care 'professionals' expecting access to medical records grew rapidly and various Government departments demanded access to medical records as a right.

The introduction of computerised records has dramatically increased the size of this problem. When medical notes were kept on paper and stored in files it was relatively easy for a doctor to deny access to official snoops (who might have difficulty in deciphering what was written even if they did manage to obtain access). When I was a general practitioner I remember a visitor from the Government arriving and announcing that he was going to remove all the medical records from my office so that they could be studied by bureaucrats. When I objected he pointed out that the paper on which the records were written belonged to the Government. I countered by pointing out that the ink was mine. I told him that he could take the paper but that he would have to leave the ink behind. He left confused and unhappy but empty-handed. But it is difficult, if not impossible to defend the principle of confidentiality now that medical records are stored on computers.

In practical terms anything a patient tells a doctor must, these days, be regarded as being in the public domain. Nurses, social workers, administrators, policemen, court officials, computer operators, typists, secretaries and people just passing by will have access to your private medical records. So many people will able to find out what diseases you have had and what secrets you have shared with your doctor that you must assume that everyone in the world will, if they so desire, know everything there is to know about you. The police, of course, have about as much respect for the concept of 'confidentiality' as they have for 'freedom' or 'justice'.

29

These days, thanks to the politicians, doctors can get into serious trouble (and be sent to prison) for not killing patients and for not telling the authorities things they were told in confidence by their patients.

30

Doctors exist only for two reasons: to look after people who have acquired a disease, and to prevent healthy people from falling ill. That's it. The rest is unimportant.

But today's medical profession has been bribed by drug companies, bullied by, and overwhelmed by bureaucrats and social workers, and forced by politicians to abandon most of their ethical principles (including, for example, the traditional principle of confidentiality). Through the weakness of their leaders, doctors have been turned into ethically impoverished mercenaries. Principles should be indigestible but the modern medical profession has swallowed its principles without hesitation or regret.

It is, perhaps, hardly surprising that most doctors now hate their jobs and regard them as little more than a way of making money. Many doctors would prefer to do something else for a living — if they could find something as lucrative. Vocation has been abandoned and replaced by expediency.

31

Medicine used to be a proud and independent profession. Sadly, much of the modern medical profession is now little more than a marketing arm for the pharmaceutical industry and a snitch service for the government. And things are likely to get worse rather than better.

32

The power of the government and of large corporations is these days so great that you cannot believe anything you see, hear or read on medical matters which is published or broadcast by a mainstream publisher or broadcaster.

33

To look after your health properly — and to reduce your chances of needing a doctor — you need access to information which you know you can trust.

But that's not easy.

Much of the medical information in magazines or newspapers has been reprinted directly from press releases produced by drug companies, or written by journalists who know far less about health care than you do. Very few publications, radio stations or television stations have on their staff anyone capable of interpreting a clinical trial properly or of reading a scientific paper and spotting the holes in it. And the so-called experts they consult are frequently paid not by the media but by drug companies. The mainstream media is dominated by government and drug company spokesmen and women. On radio and television the spokesman you hear advocating vaccines or some new wonder drug will probably be receiving payments from drug companies. Even books published by mainstream publishers are suspect, with some published with the aid of advance orders from drug companies or the meat industry. There are even doctors who are paid to write letters to newspapers promoting or defending certain foodstuffs or drug therapies.

34

Modern journalists seem to have very little knowledge of the things they write about. Here is one of dozens of examples I could give.

In July 2006, newspapers ran a story about hair dyes causing cancer.

'Dying hair increases cancer risk' screamed one headline. 'Using hair dye can increase the chance of developing cancer, new research suggests.' said another.

The newspapers described this story as though it was hot news.

It wasn't.

I devoted several pages to the problems of cancer caused by hair dyes in a book called *Face Values* which was published in 1981.

35

Like many doctors who dare to question the views and actions of the medical establishment I have repeatedly found that mainstream journalists (whether they work in print or are broadcasters) will rarely dare to publish views (however well-supported by the facts) which question the accepted official line.

For example, when a researcher for a TV programme called to ask me whether I thought drugs given for patients with cancer were worthwhile I told him that I could provide evidence showing that the use of such drugs is a waste of time and money, and that the real way to tackle cancer is to boost the patient's immune system. I explained that many anti-cancer drugs do the opposite. The researcher was enthusiastic but I predicted that the programme's editors and producers would not dare include my point of view. My prediction proved entirely accurate.

Similar things happen on a regular basis. My conclusion is that journalists are rarely willing to risk upsetting politicians or large, powerful industries. I have been contacted many, many times by researchers wanting to know if I would help with programmes about the dangers of meat, the hazards of prescription drugs, the safety of vaccinations and the value of vivisection. Occasionally the programmes have been made. Invitations for me to take part have always been withdrawn.

36

Advertisements for my book *How To Stop Your Doctor Killing You* were banned on the grounds that my claim that 'the person most likely to kill you is not a murderer or a drunken motorist but your doctor' was unfair to doctors.

Unfair?

In the UK each year:

* around 859 people are murdered
* around 2663 people are killed in road accidents

And how many patients are killed by doctors? At a conservative estimate the figure is well over 20,000. The official figures show that there 980,000 'patient safety incidents' in the National Health Service hospitals in 2004, and that over 2,000 patients died because of cock- ups. These are the official figures and are an absurd under-estimate of the real size of the problem. No one working in the NHS (whether a doctor, nurse or administrator) is likely to report a side effect or error unless they feel they have to. The American style enthusiasm for litigation is the reason for this shyness.

The advertisement was banned by a small private organisation called the Advertising Standards Authority (the ASA).

Where, you are no doubt asking, does the ASA get its money from?

Mainly from large companies.

Possibly including drug companies.

37

The ASA also banned an advertisement which simply invited readers to visit my website to study the facts about animal experiments. The evidence supporting the advertisement was readily available on my website and included evidence given to the House of Lords.

The ASA claimed to have received one complaint (which may have been from a vivisector or vivisection supporter). They refused to identify the complainant.

The ASA's report criticising the advertisement is bizarre. They were advised to study the evidence on my website. In their report they admitted that they had viewed some of the content (they actually use the word 'some') but were unable to find what they were looking for.

So they decided that the advertisement was misleading and banned it.

The ASA seems to me to be riding roughshod over my fundamental rights as an individual, an author and an advertiser in the interests of protecting large, international industries which can quite well look after themselves.

38

Some people think that the ASA is more concerned with protecting big business than the interests of consumers.

Last year the organisation took no action at all against the five advertisements which had caused the most offence to ordinary consumers.

Five advertisements which had between them attracted more than 3,600 angry complaints were left untouched by the ASA All these advertisements had been placed by large companies.

On the other hand the ASA has consistently ruled against advertisements placed by anti-vivisectors — even though only one complaint may have been received.

For example, when the Research Defence Society (an organisation set up and funded to defend vivisection) complained about two antivivisection leaflets of mine, the ASA quickly banned them. Amazingly, one of the people on the ASA committee which banned the leaflets was the vice chairman of L'Oreal (UK) Ltd, a large cosmetics company which has in the past been criticised by anti-vivisectors for its use of ingredients tested by means of animal experiments.

Coleman's 9th Law Of Medicine

Doctors and nurses know little or nothing about staying healthy. In particular, doctors and nurses know nothing useful about food, diet and healthy eating. (Sadly, the same is true of nutritionists and dieticians).

1

Doctors have never taken much interest in preventive medicine. This, I'm afraid, is because they have little (or, rather, no) financial interest in keeping their patients healthy. Except in China (where doctors were once paid only for as long as their patients stayed well) doctors have always earned their money out of diagnosing and curing illness. When you earn money out of making people healthy when they are ill, keeping them healthy makes no financial sense at all. And, however incompetent some doctors may be, none of them are entirely stupid.

2

During the last few hundred years we have changed our world much faster than our bodies have managed to evolve. That's why we suffer so much from stress-related diseases. We still have bodies designed to cope with the sort of threat posed by sabre toothed tigers but we live in a world where our stresses come in brown envelopes and land on our doormats every day.

Similarly, we have changed the food we eat faster than our bodies have been able to adapt

We were designed (or slowly evolved) for a very different type of diet to the one most of us eat today. We were designed for a diet based on fruits and vegetables, supplemented occasionally with a small amount of lean meat. We weren't designed to eat vast quantities of fatty meat, we weren't designed to drink milk taken from another animal (and meant for its young) and we weren't designed to eat grains.

Around 99.99% of our genetic material was formed when we were eating the sort of diet for which we were designed.

But now most of us live on fatty meat, milky foods and cereals.

There were 100,000 generations of humans known as hunter-gatherers (living on fruits and vegetables they gathered and animals they occasionally managed to kill) and 500 generations dependent on agriculture (living on food grown on farms and animals reared in captivity).

There have been just ten generations of humans since the onset of the industrial age and just two generations have grown up with highly processed fast, junk food.

Knowing all this it is hardly surprising that we are most of us ill most of the time.

3

'Leave your drugs in the chemist's pot if you can heal your patient with food.'

Hippocrates, 5th century BC

4

Obesity is now endemic in most Western countries. And type 2 diabetes (also known as maturity onset diabetes) is often a consequence of obesity. And yet most doctors do little or nothing either to help their patients to lose weight or to diagnose type 2 diabetes. It has, for example, been reliably estimated that in some countries about a quarter of the people who have diabetes do not know that they have diabetes. Since diabetes can cause numerous health problems — and can kill — this is clearly a serious problem. In Britain, for example, it is estimated that around 500,000 women have diabetes but don't know it.

When diabetes is diagnosed the doctor's usual response is to reach for a prescription pad and prescribe one of the potentially hazardous drugs promoted for the purpose.

In fact, most patients could control their diabetes (and protect themselves from health problems) by changing their diet (cutting out junk foods) and losing excess weight.

But prescribing a pill is easier than giving advice. And taking a pill is easier than cutting down on cream cakes.

5

Our ancestors ate raw fruits, nuts, seeds, wild game (low in fat) and hundreds of different types of plant.

A broad range of plants gives a wide range of vitamins and minerals and other secondary plant compounds. Such a diet helps to keep us healthy when we are well and to heal us when we are not.

We need fresh, organic fruit and vegetables in good quantities but these days we eat very few plants. We eat the plants which farmers find easy to grow and which are most profitable. Things are made infinitely worse by the fact that modern methods of farming rely on chemical intervention. And some of the chemicals are carcinogenic.

To stay healthy most of us need supplements. They help but they are nowhere near as good as a healthy, natural diet.

6

Is it a coincidence that when gorillas are brought into captivity and fed on the sort of diet we think they should eat (not dissimilar, of course, from the sort of diet we eat ourselves) they too develop heart disease, ulcerative colitis and high cholesterol levels — problems they don't suffer from in the wild? Given the opportunity to become couch potatoes, baboons will jump at the idea. The Masai Mara National Reserve on the Serengeti Plains of Kenya has baboons who traditionally pick and choose their diet from everything available. But as the Park has grown it has inevitably attracted tourists, hotels and rubbish. Within a few years of the first waste dump being formed the baboons found that they could just lie around until the waste lorry arrived and then binge on high fat, high protein, high sugar leftovers. The baboons feeding like this grow faster, reach puberty earlier and weigh more. But their cholesterol levels have shot up and they get diabetes and chronic heart disease.

In North America the same thing happens to wild bears who hang around waste dumps and car parks in places such as the Yosemite National Park. They become obese and ill. And they also become mentally disturbed; showing signs of confusion and becoming increasingly violent.

Is it coincidence that the hunter-gatherer societies which still exist in the world's few wild, remote areas have far less cancer, heart disease, diabetes and osteoporosis? They may die falling from trees or being eaten by wild animals but they don't die from the sort of diseases which cripple and kill us. Time and time again anthropologists have observed that as native societies abandon their traditional hunter-gatherer lifestyle so their health deteriorates.

Today, we are like captive cows and sheep, falling ill because they can no longer choose a varied diet but must rely on what the farmers choose to offer.

7

The drug industry has efficiently persuaded us that medicine and food are separate things. When we think of 'medicine' we are encouraged to think of 'drugs'. (To many people the words 'medicine' and 'drug' have become interchangeable.)

The drug industry has turned natural compounds into drugs, making them more powerful and more dangerous and it has patented new chemical compounds and then promoted them with far more enthusiasm than scientific sense. Drug companies have even patented traditional herbal products.

The drug companies have encouraged us to believe that when we are ill we must take something to rid ourselves of our symptoms. It's all about money.

8

There are 76 million cases of food-related infectious illnesses in the United States of America every year — with around 5,000 deaths.

Figures for other countries are probably similar. These figures are probably on the low side since it seems likely that many people who have short-lived illnesses do not bother to report them to anyone. (Who would you tell if you didn't need to call the doctor? And how many doctors bother to report such illnesses to their government anyway?)

Illnesses caused by drinking contaminated water do not count for these figures since water is not regarded as a food. If water borne contamination (and other forms of contamination) were added the total number of incidents of food-related infectious illness in the USA would exceed 200,000,000 cases a year. That, believe me, is a lot of vomit and a lot of diarrhoea.

Many of these problems are caused by the contamination of food with bacteria, viruses and other organisms. Since human and animal waste is widely used in animal feed this is hardly surprising. (In the autumn of 1999 French farmers were vilified for feeding human waste to their animals. This was all part of a political game. The disgusting practice of feeding faeces to animals is widespread and is certainly not confined to France.)

9

Attempts to control the dramatically increasing problem of food related illness have been futile. Governments everywhere are nervous about upsetting the powerful food industry and even more nervous about upsetting farmers.

Of course, food which is contaminated with infective organisms isn't the only reason why people are falling ill these days. If cases of cancer, heart disease and other diseases caused by diet were added the numbers involved would be much more dramatic. There is no absolutely no doubt that at least a third of all cancers are caused by food. (Recent research suggests that up to 70% of human cancers may be triggered by chemicals released during the breakdown of food.) And there are strong links between specific foods and most other major killers too. (Important medical and scientific evidence appears in my book Food for Thought.)

10

In an attempt to stay healthy most of us want to eat nutritious, healthy food that tastes good and does us good. We want to be able to pay a fair price for food that contains natural ingredients and, ideally, no chemical residues. If the food we are buying contains additives we would like to know what they are.

In order to make sure that we do our best to eat healthily we naturally put a lot of faith in the labels used to describe the food we eat.

Our faith is misplaced.

Encouraged and supported by governments food companies lie, lie and lie again. Ordinary, everyday words such as 'fresh', 'natural', 'wholesome' and 'nutritious' are virtually meaningless. If the American Government has its way the word 'organic' will soon be entirely meaningless too.

We all put our faith in labels — and our trust in the people who sell us food. But our faith and our trust are misplaced. Food companies are aware of our desire for genuinely good food and so they employ clever advertising and marketing 'spin doctors' to help disguise the way that the food they sell us is adulterated by behind-the-scene chemists. Here are some of the ways food companies defraud us:

Spring water
The phrase can be used to describe water that has been taken out of a tap.

Meat
The word 'meat' can be used to describe anything that comes from an animal — from the tip of its nose to the tip of its tail. Scraps of meat blasted off the bones are counted, as are bits of faeces clinging to tissues.

Farmfresh and Farmhouse
Utterly meaningless words. The foods described in this way can be produced in factories from animals or birds (such as hens) kept in battery cages.

Fresh

This means whatever the food company wants it to mean.

GM Free
If you think that a 'GM Free' label means that food doesn't contain genetically modified food you would be wrong. The rules mean that food can contain a small quantity of genetically modified food and yet be described as not containing genetically modified food. Since the whole point with genetically engineered food is that a small amount may induce cancer (there is no evidence that it does and no evidence that it doesn't) this is dangerous and absurd. Incidentally, studies on genetically engineered cotton have created real concerns. In New Zealand farmers found that thousands of sheep had died after grazing on land where genetically engineered cotton had been grown. Another report showed that workers who picked genetically engineered cotton suffered severe skin eruptions. What will genetically engineered food do to anyone who eats it? I haven't got the foggiest notion. And nor, I suspect, has anyone else.

Steak
This implies that the item is a solid piece of flesh. But this isn't necessarily so. 'Steaks' can be built up using scraps and flakes of flesh.

Low fat
This doesn't mean anything since there are no legal rules defining what 'low fat' means.
This doesn't mean anything either. Nor does Extra Lean. (Nor, for that matter, Extra Extra Lean.) A product described as 'lean' may sound as though it

contains little fat but it can be just as fatty as any other product.

Flavour
Don't make the mistake of assuming that the phrase 'banana flavour' implies that the food you are buying has anything to do with bananas. The flavour may be made in a laboratory from chemicals.

Free Range
This doesn't necessarily mean that the hens (or other creatures) range free. It can mean that a vast number of creatures share limited access to a very limited outdoor space. Free-range chickens are merely chickens who are technically allowed to stretch their legs. Most are fed on mass produced pellets and never see a hay barn or a blade of grass. Chemicals may be added to the feed in order to try to improve the appearance of the yolks — and in order to keep the hens alive in their unnatural 'free range' conditions. (If you and ten thousand other people lived in one room with a door into a carpet sized garden would you describe yourself as 'free range'?)

Brown bread
Sounds wholesome but it can be white bread which has been dyed brown.

Natural
This word doesn't mean anything when applied to food. Or, rather, it means whatever the food manufacturer wants it to mean.

Smoked

If you think your smoked bacon has been smoked you are probably being naive. Your bacon may well have been pumped up with an artificial smoke flavour liquid.

Country Fresh Eggs
The hens are probably kept in a battery but the battery may be in the country. The word 'fresh' means whatever the food company wants it to mean.

Nutritious
This doesn't mean anything at all. A food company could happily package pig faeces and label it 'nutritious'.

How do food companies get away with all this deceit?

Largely, I'm afraid, because most people don't bother to complain.

11

The quality and quantity of the food we eat is vitally important for the preservation of our good health.

If you eat fatty food, full of chemicals and preservatives, you will be far more likely to develop and die of cancer or heart disease than if you eat a low fat, high fibre diet in which fruit and vegetables play a major part.

If doctors told their patients the truth about food most of the world's drug companies would virtually disappear within months. The market for heart drugs, high blood pressure drugs, anti-cancer drugs and so on would fall through the floor. Drug companies would be struggling along side-by-side with the buggy whip manufacturers.

And yet the advice about nutrition given to patients by doctors, nurses, nutritionists and dieticians is often appalling and frequently lethal. The food served in hospitals (where people are, it can safely be assumed, at their weakest and at their greatest need of wholesome, nutritious food) is almost universally inedible and customarily harmful to the patient. The food produced for patients is nothing more than unwholesome stodge, full of calories and fat and devoid of vitamins. You're more likely to find salmonella or staphylococci in a plateful of hospital food than you are to find an antioxidant.

12

There is a single food that causes most illness (and which causes as many deaths and as much illness as tobacco). It is a food which has been proven time and time again to cause cancer of the breast, cancer of the prostate, cancer of the bowel, many other types of cancer and numerous other disorders including asthma, heart disease, constipation, high blood pressure, osteoporosis and rheumatoid arthritis. It is a food which most people eat at least once every day. And it is a food which governments know is potentially lethal. But the truth about this deadly food is suppressed for purely commercial reasons. Governments (and the medical profession) say nothing because the people selling the food have too much power and too much money.

The name of the food is meat. The United States Surgeon General's Report called 'Nutrition and Health' said: 'In one international correlational study...a positive association was observed between total protein and animal protein and breast, colon, prostate, renal and endometrial cancers.'

It is, I believe, the fat in meat which is the most significant cause of cancer. The fat in meat isn't just the white stuff that is easy to cut off. The fat is spread throughout the meat and is invisible to the naked eye.

13

The fat in meat is particularly likely to cause cancer because the chemicals with which animals are fed accumulate in the fat. Breast cancer is a particular risk because breast tissue contains a considerable amount of fatty tissue. The carcinogenic chemicals fed to animals accumulate in the animal's fatty tissues. When the fatty meat is eaten the carcinogenic chemicals easily accumulate in the parts of the human body with the most fat.

14

All sorts of people have produced all sorts of explanations for the dramatic rise in breast cancer in recent years. The use of talcum powder and the wearing of bras have both been blamed. Other scientists claimed that it is the fact that so many women now work nights — with the result that their hormones are disrupted.

The real answer is much simpler, far more obvious and eminently easy to prove. Unfortunately, it is also inconvenient for the governments and a huge industry.

The truth is that breast cancer is rocketing (as are so many other cancers) because of chemical toxins in the fatty meat we eat. Clear scientific evidence shows that women who eat lots of fat, and/or eat lots of meat, are more likely to get breast cancer. It really is that simple.

15

The incidence of breast cancer among Japanese women was low when they ate a traditional Japanese diet (which contains very little meat). When Japanese women started eating fatty hamburgers (food which I long ago christened harmburgers) the incidence of breast cancer rocketed.

16

Modern regulations allow farmers, meat processors, packers and food companies selling meat to mislead their consumers in a way that would probably startle people in other industries. The word 'meat' can include the head, feet, rectum (full or empty), spinal cord and tail of an animal. The term 'meat product' can include the eyeballs and the nose. A package which is labelled as pure beef may include fat, rind, gristle and skin. It is commonplace for sausages to include ground up tonsils, fat, bone, cartilage and intestines (with or without the contents). The people selling meat and meat products use flavourings and colourings to disguise what they are selling. Faecal matter is an advantage because it adds extra weight. Water and polyphosphates are injected into an animal's dead body at high pressure in order to increase the weight of the animal and the profit to the farmer.

17

There is plenty of evidence proving that meat causes cancer (there are summaries of 26 scientific papers relating meat to cancer in my book *Food for Thought* and on my websites www.vernoncoleman.com and www.vernoncoleman.co.uk) but, despite this, there are many doctors, dieticians and nutritionists around who still don't seem to understand the importance of this link. Despite the firm evidence showing that meat causes cancer the majority of hospitals still serve their patients (and staff) meals which are built around meat. We think it strange that just a relatively few years ago patients and staff in hospitals were allowed to smoke on the wards but in a few years' time our descendants will surely regard it as just as odd that hospitals should serve meat to people entrusted to their care. Any nutritionist, dietician, cookery writer or chef who advocates eating meat is woefully ignorant about food and health, in the pay of the meat industry or a plain old-fashioned psychopath who likes killing people and should be doing something else for a living. This is beyond argument. It is as absurd and as indefensible for a chef, nutritionist or dietician to recommend eating meat as part of a healthy diet as it would be for a doctor to recommend smoking as part of a healthy lifestyle.

18

Meat dishes in restaurants should carry exactly the same sort of Government health warning as packets of cigarettes. Meat on sale in butchers' shops should carry the same warning. If one makes a judgement objectively, based purely on the available scientific evidence, chefs who promote meat eating should be arrested and charged with manslaughter and parents who give their children meat to eat should be charged with negligence. (Children are still developing until the age of about 12 and young immune systems and livers are less able to get rid of contaminants.)

19

The list of diseases known to be associated with meat, or to be commoner among meat eaters, looks like the index of a medical textbook.

Anaemia, appendicitis, arthritis, breast cancer, cancer of the colon, cancer of the prostate, constipation, diabetes, gall stones, gout, high blood pressure, indigestion, obesity, piles, strokes and varicose veins are just some of the well-known disorders which are more likely to affect meat eaters than vegetarians.

There is too, the problem of the adrenalin in meat. When animals are killed they are inevitably terrified. They have a good deal of adrenalin running through their veins. When the animal is eaten the person who eats the animal consumes that adrenalin. What are the consequences of this? No one knows.

20

Avoiding meat is one of the best and simplest ways to cut down your fat consumption. When animal fat is metabolised in the body it produces damaging free radicals which help cause cancer, cardiovascular disease and ageing.

21

Those who eat beef are, in my view, foolishly exposing themselves to the risk of contracting the horrifying human version of Mad Cow Disease.

22

To all these hazards must be added the fact that if you eat meat you will be consuming any hormones, drugs and other chemicals which may have been fed to the animals before they were killed.

No one knows precisely what effect eating the hormones in meat is likely to have on your health. But the risk is there and I think it's a big one.

And there are other hazards. Some farmers use tranquillisers to keep animals calm. Others routinely use antibiotics so that their animals do not develop infections — and to boost the rate at which they put on weight. In America over half of all antibiotics are fed to animals and I don't think it is any coincidence that the percentage of staphylococci infections resistant to penicillin went up from 13% in 1960 to 91 % in 1988. Animals which are lucky enough to spend some of their time out of doors eating grass will often eat grass which has been sprayed with all sorts of toxic and carcinogenic chemicals.

23

The link between fat, fatty meat and cancer is not new. But Western Governments have suppressed the truth so effectively that it was only in 2005 that newspapers acknowledged the link. One newspaper reported this 'discovery' with the front page headline: 'Chips Can Increase The Risk Of Breast Cancer'. The same newspaper article also seemed astonished to be able to report that women who are overweight are more at risk of developing breast cancer. They reported that women between the ages of 18 and 30 who lost 10lb in weight cut their chances of developing breast cancer before the age of 50 by 65% and that the women who benefited most were the women who had a mutation in the gene which is recognised to increase the risk of breast cancer. (It is, of course, these women who are usually offered the option of having their breasts removed — a savage and pointless operation which is one of the most fashionable currently offered to patients. See Coleman's 7th Law Of Medicine.)

24

The healthiness of a vegetarian diet is perhaps shown most dramatically by the fact that lifelong vegetarians visit hospitals 22% less often than meat eaters — and for shorter stays.

Vegetarians tend to be fitter than meat eaters — as well as healthier — and many of the world's most successful athletes (particularly those who specialise in endurance events) follow a strictly vegetarian diet.

25

There are all sorts of old-fashioned myths about eating meat. For example, it used to be claimed that people who didn't eat meat would be short of protein. That is now known to be absolute nonsense. And it is equally untrue that if you don't eat meat your diet will be deficient in essential vitamins or minerals. Meat contains absolutely nothing — no protein, vitamins or minerals — that your body cannot obtain perfectly happily from a vegetarian diet.

26

The Atkins diet (which I have attacked ever since it first became popular — I've always thought that 'give grease a chance' would have been a good slogan for it) has acquired many keen followers and its emphasis on eating meat made it very popular with the meat industry. At one point around 20 million people around the world were thought to be on this high fat diet. Sadly for those individuals the body needs carbohydrates and without them it takes what it needs from stores in the muscles and liver. It is inevitable that problems will develop. The side effects known to be associated with the Atkins diet include bowel problems, muscle weakness and headaches. Heaven knows what the long-term effects might be. I suspect that long before all the harmful effects are identified lawsuits from unhappy dieters will have consigned the Atkins diet to the graveyard wherein so many other crazy and unhealthy diets now reside.

27

Why don't governments stop people eating meat?

For the same reason that they don't put much effort into stopping people smoking and drinking too much alcohol. They want the taxes made by the manufacturers of these products (and, in many cases, the bribes offered by the manufacturers lobbyists) and they don't want their citizens to live too long anyway. Your government wants you dead before you become an expensive drag on society, retiring, failing to work and pay taxes, claiming a pension and using up expensive health services. Doctors, to their everlasting shame, do nothing so spread the truth.

28

Astonishingly, some doctors actively encourage their patients to eat meat.

After reading in the national press that a doctor in England was alleged to be 'prescribing rump steak and pork chops' to his patients I wrote to the General Medical Council (the organisation which regulates and registers doctors in the United Kingdom) asking them to investigate. There is, I pointed out, ample evidence available to show that meat causes cancer. (From the newspaper reports, I gathered that the doctor's activities were being encouraged by the meat industry)

I offered to provide the General Medical Council with over 20 scientific papers, published in reputable journals (including the *International Journal of Cancer, New England Journal of Medicine, Cancer Research, British Journal of Cancer, Cancer, British Medical Journal*) showing that eating meat causes cancer. I also pointed out that the United States Surgeon General has reported links between meat eating and cancer. I suggested to the General Medical Council that this was a matter of significant public interest and should be attended to without delay.

I was not in the slightest bit surprised to receive a letter from the General Medical Council dismissing my complaint. 'We have carefully considered the information you provided...however, we have decided that this is not a matter that justifies action by us. The issue you have mentioned does not appear to have any bearing on the doctor's ability to practise medicine and does not breach our guidance.'

So, according to the General Medical Council, it is perfectly acceptable for a doctor to recommend that his patients eat food that may give them cancer.

29

Spreading the truth about meat isn't easy.

Advertisements for my book *Food for Thought* (which contains scientific evidence showing that meat causes cancer) have, naturally, been banned by the Advertising Standards Authority. Even a British satirical magazine called *Private Eye* (which has created and cultivated an image for taking a tough attitude to the establishment and which likes to give the impression that it is fearless and carefree) refused to accept an advertisement for my book *Food for Thought* which included the words 'meat causes cancer'.

30

The risks associated with eating meat are generally wildly underestimated by both patients and doctors. But patients and doctors are poor at assessing risks. I know people who smoke but who won't fly because they consider air travel too dangerous. (Their risk of contracting a deadly disease through smoking is massively greater than their risk of dying in an aeroplane crash). I know people who ride motorbikes but who won't use mobile phones. (I was one of the first to draw attention to the possible risks associated with mobile phone use — particularly for children — but even I don't think that mobile phones are as dangerous as riding motor bikes). And I know people who regularly take sleeping tablets but who are severely disapproving of others who have a whisky night cap to help them sleep. (A tot of whisky at bedtime is far less likely to produce serious addiction and other problems than the regular use of sleeping tablets.)

31

I hope you've got the message about meat now. I've rather laboured the point because the pro-meat lobby has spent zillions flogging its death-inducing product and I know I have a lot of misinformation to counteract The industry selling meat is extremely powerful and has supported and created numerous campaigns to sell its product.

32

Research into whether mobile phones cause brain cancer would be easy to organise. One way is to find a few thousand people with brain tumours and check out which side of their head the tumour is on. Then ask them whether they are right or left-handed. Alternatively, it would be easy to find out if the number of brain tumours has increased since phones became popular. Instead, researchers conducting experiments to assess the safety of mobile telephones have used mice.

The truth is that the mobile phone industry is conducting the world's largest biological experiment — with 1.3 billion users. I don't believe anyone really knows what will happen. Governments do and say nothing to halt the spread the sale of mobile telephones because they need the taxes paid by the manufacturers and users of these products.

Astonishingly (and frighteningly) a quarter of 7-10 year old children already have a mobile phone and phone companies are now designing special mobile phones for young children (America's *Business Week* magazine called them 'cell phones for the sand lot') which are simpler to use for those who haven't yet mastered such intricacies as the alphabet. (A growing percentage of adults, blessed with illiteracy thanks to modern education policies might welcome such phones too.)

33

Food experts are often 'bought' by the big food companies. This is the only way to explain the fact many so-called experts seem to understand less about food, health and disease than the average kitchen sink Many organisations which describe themselves as 'independent', and which have wonderfully grand sounding names, are in fact nothing more than lobby groups set up and funded by large food companies. It is this funding which explains why so many seemingly sane sounding experts, centres, institutes, forums and foundations pontificate in public about just how good hamburgers and sugar coated cereals are for us. It is these self-appointed experts and guardians who are likely to announce (without any apparent embarrassment) that we need to do research to discover the causes of obesity and that there are no known links between food and cancer.

34

Our eating habits have been manipulated so that we satisfy our short-term eating goals. We are encouraged to give in to temptation and to suppress our natural instincts. We don't eat to stay healthy or to become healthy, but for kicks. Sweet things attract us because of the energy kick they give. Fatty food tastes good. Chocolate contains fat, sugar and a bitter stimulant that is addictive. Processed foods don't provide anything we really need other than instant energy. The problem is that the food industry gives us not what we need but what we want. As with tobacco, alcohol and drugs we get hooked on products that seem to ease the psychological problems which have been created by our lifestyle. And, of course, though these products may produce short-term solutions they create long-term problems of their own.

35

There is clear evidence to show that how much food you eat is just as important as what you eat. Eating less can lead to a longer life.

A team from the Louisiana State University in the USA monitored a group of 48 overweight men and women aged between 25 and 50 years. A quarter of them were put on a diet containing 25% fewer calories than they would be expected to eat for their age and weight. Another quarter had their calorie intake reduced by 12.5% and were also put on a strict exercise regime. A third group stuck to a very strict diet of just 890 calories a day. Finally, the last group was placed on a diet which would enable them to maintain their weight.

The results showed that the volunteers on the fewest calories lost, on average, 14% of their body weight during the six months. The other calorie-restricted dieters lost 10% of their body weight. All the volunteers who cut down their calories showed a fall in their average body temperature and showed reduced fasting insulin levels — both figures which are linked to longevity. The rate at which their DNA decayed also slowed. This is important because decaying DNA increases the chances of mutations and degenerative diseases developing, and producing problems such as cancer.

Other research has shown that people who eat less also have healthier hearts.

Researchers believe that cutting calories reduces the production of free radicals, the toxic particles which are difficult for the body to get rid of. The message is simple: eat less, live longer.

If you eat like a bird you'll live as long as an elephant.

So why don't doctors and dieticians warn patients of this?

Simple.

Where's the profit?

36

Thousands of people pay a premium to eat organic food in the belief that what they are eating has not been sprayed with poisonous chemicals.

Oh dear.

In many parts of the world the fact that a food is labelled 'organic' does not necessarily mean that it has not been sprayed with chemicals. It means only that it has (or may have been) sprayed with *approved* chemicals. Having seen the rapid growth in the size of the market for organic food (sales in America in 1980 were worth less than £100 million but in 2003 they were worth £5 billion) American farmers and food manufacturers have insisted that the standards be lowered and the rules changed.

How toxic are the approved chemicals?

Good question.

Your guess is undoubtedly just as good as mine. And since the rules vary from country to country our guesses are as good as anyone else's.

The only sure way to make sure that you eat truly organic food is to grow it yourself.

And to make sure that you don't spray your crop or add chemicals to the soil.

37

There is one form of preventive medicine with which doctors and nurses are very well acquainted: most are enthusiastic about vaccines.

Are they right to be so? Should you have your child vaccinated? Who should you believe about vaccination? The Government? The drug companies? The medical establishment? Television?

For over thirty years I have been warning about the potential problems associated with vaccines. I have, during that time, provided a considerable amount of proof showing that vaccination programmes often do more harm than good. To be precise, I believe that the amount of illness and the number of deaths caused by vaccinations far exceeds the amount of serious illness and the number of deaths caused by the diseases against which the vaccinations are supposed to offer protection. The most significant known facts about vaccines are that they can cause brain damage and they can kill. The evidence shows that some vaccines kill and injure far more people than the diseases the vaccines are given to protect against.

This isn't theory or supposition. It is fact.

Since the late 1970s the British Government has quietly handed out tens of thousands of pounds in damages to parents of children suffering from brain damage caused by vaccines.

38

I also believe, and have believed for many years, that autism is caused by vaccination.

The word autism is said to be used, like the word cancer, as an umbrella term for a range of different problems. Patients with autism are said to have development disorders which affect their ability to interact socially and to communicate with other people though this is a fairly recent interpretation and the word does seem to be used as a catch-all for a whole range of problems. (In one medical dictionary on my shelf autism is defined as 'morbid self-absorption'.) These days, I suspect that the word is used more as a dustbin word rather than an umbrella word. It helps the profession appear to know what is the matter when they don't and, at the same time, it enables them to avoid taking any responsibility for what has happened. The word is used to describe almost any symptoms which doctors cannot explain. Autism can be anything from a mild behavioural problem to severe brain damage.

Social workers and other professional lightweights play the game because it enables them to build well-funded empires around the 'care' of autistic patients. For governments it is, of course, a lot cheaper to provide 'care' for autistic patients than to acknowledge that these children have been made ill by the official vaccination policy and should have been provided with vast amounts of compensation.

I believe that the epidemiological evidence supports this hypothesis. The number of children being diagnosed as suffering from autism has rocketed as the number of children being vaccinated has rocketed. Once rare (in the 1990s it was generally accepted that autism affected no more than 4 or 5 people in every 10,000), it is now officially claimed that it affects more than one in 100 children in Britain. (Some experts claim that the real figure is much higher than this.) Figures in other countries show that the incidence of autism is rising in all developed countries. How anyone can deny the possibility of a link between vaccination and autism is quite beyond me. The epidemiological evidence is overwhelming. If vaccines are known to cause brain damage isn't it logical to assume that they can also cause the disease which is known as autism but which would, I believe, be more properly and honestly known as brain damage? I have been suggesting that there is a link between 'autism' and vaccination for decades and no one has yet discredited my theories. A vast number of the children currently being diagnosed as 'autistic' are, without a doubt, actually suffering from various levels of brain damage caused by vaccines. Doctors and drug companies and politicians much prefer to talk about autism rather than brain damage because the former suggests a natural disease while the latter suggests that there may be an external cause. Innocent and desperate parents collude with this nonsense because they prefer to describe their children as autistic rather than as brain damaged.

39

The drug companies (and the doctors, hospitals and politicians who support them) all claim that there is no link between autism and vaccination. (But then they would, wouldn't they?). They claim that there is no convincing scientific evidence proving a link between the two. (On the other hand there is no convincing scientific evidence disproving a link between vaccination and autism.)

When a research project was set up to investigate the link, drug companies applied to a London court for an injunction to stop the research.

Now why would they do that?

I really can't imagine.

40

If children scream or are unusually quiet or show other unusual signs after a vaccination then there is, I suspect, a real chance that they will develop autism. Sadly, of course, it is too late to do anything about it by then.

41

As the years have gone by the number of vaccines available has increased steadily. Modern American children now receive around thirty vaccinations by the time they go to school.

A decade or two ago the only vaccines available were against a relatively small number of diseases including smallpox, tuberculosis, polio, cholera, diphtheria, tetanus and whooping cough. Today, the number of available vaccines seems to grow almost weekly. In the past vaccines were produced against major killer diseases. Today vaccines are produced against diseases such as measles, mumps and chickenpox which have traditionally been regarded as relatively benign inconveniences of childhood.

The death rate from measles had dropped dramatically decades before the vaccine against measles was introduced. Today, despite (or, perhaps, because of) the widespread use of the vaccine, the incidence of measles is rising again.

42

In attempts to persuade parents to have their children vaccinated against measles governments and doctors around the world have thought up an apparently unending — and hysterical — series of scare campaigns. Now that there is a vaccine against it, measles has, by a strange coincidence, stopped being an annoying childhood disease and has, instead, become a deadly killer.

43

Scares designed to encourage parents to have their children vaccinated often consist of claiming that a major epidemic is just around the corner and that only vaccination can offer protection. I have lost count of the number whooping cough epidemics which governments have wrongly forecast. Governments and their advisers are either unbelievably stupid or else they are deliberately lying to help boost drug company profits.

44

Countless scientists around the world have spent vast fortunes trying to create a vaccine against AIDS (in view of the fact that AIDS may not exist they may find this trickier than expected).

And scientists have apparently developed a banana vaccine by creating genetically engineered banana plants. There are plans to develop bananas which 'protect' those who eat them against hepatitis B, measles, yellow fever and poliomyelitis.

Other scientists have developed a genetically engineered potato which it may be possible to use as a vaccine against cholera. The active part of the potato remains active during the process of cooking and so a portion of genetically engineered chips could soon be a vaccine against cholera.

I promise you I am not making this up.

You will not be surprised to hear that I would not knowingly consume any fruit or vegetable that had been genetically modified — let alone one that had been modified in this obscene way.

45

Naturally, the pharmaceutical industry is constantly searching for more and more new vaccines. I have lost count of the number of times I have read of researchers working on a vaccine to prevent cancer. Every year new 'flu jabs appear on the market. There are, so I am told, vaccines in the pipeline for just about everything ranging from asthma to earache. There is even a planned genetically engineered vaccine which will provide protection against forty different diseases. The vaccine, which will contain the raw DNA of all those different diseases, will be given to newborn babies to provide them with protection for life. Oh, goody. Can't wait.

46

I don't know about you but I can no longer keep up with what is going on in the world of vaccines. I have long since given up trying to work out which vaccines are very dangerous and which are just a bit dangerous — and to whom. The only certainty is that manufacturing (and giving) vaccines is big business. The people who sell vaccines make a lot of money. And the doctors who give them (or who authorise nurses to give them on their behalf) make a lot of money too. Vaccination is a big and very profitable, industry.

47

Does anyone know what happens inside the body when all these different vaccinations are given together? Do different vaccines work with or against one another? What about the risk of interactions? Exactly how does the immune system cope when it is suddenly bombarded with so much foreign material? And what about dangerous contaminants? One anti-flu vaccine which was injected into over a million American citizens contained a cancer-causing monkey virus. And then there's the polio vaccine.

The polio vaccine is often used as an example of just how wonderful a vaccine can be.

And supporters of animal experiments claim that without animal experiments there would have never been a vaccine against poliomyelitis.

Both arguments are wrong.

The number of deaths from polio had fallen dramatically some time before the first polio vaccine was introduced. Better food, better housing cleaner water and better sanitation had all led to a fall in the incidence and significance of the disease.

In fact the evidence shows that the introduction of the vaccine led to more patients with polio rather than fewer. In Tennessee, USA, the number of poliomyelitis victims the year before vaccination became compulsory was 119, but the year after vaccination was introduced the number rose to 386. In North Carolina, the number of cases before vaccination was 78 while the number after the vaccine became compulsory rose to 313. There are similar figures for other American states.

The first breakthrough in the development of a poliomyelitis vaccine was made in 1949 with the aid of a human tissue culture. But when the first practical vaccine was prepared in the 1950s monkey kidney tissue was used because that was standard laboratory practice. Researchers didn't realise that one of the viruses commonly found in monkey kidney cells can cause cancer in humans. If human cells had been used to prepare the vaccine (as they could and should have been and as they are now) the original poliomyelitis vaccine would have been much safer.

48

How many other vaccines contain similarly dangerous ingredients? Could the constant increase in the incidence of cancer be connected to the enthusiasm for vaccination programmes which has for decades now been inspired by drug companies and governments and maintained by doctors?

49

I am an enthusiastic supporter of the principle of preventive medicine. It is usually much easier to avoid an illness than it is to treat one.

Vaccination programmes are usually sold to the public as though they are an integral part of a general preventive medicine programme. But vaccination programmes cannot truly be described as preventive medicine. They are, rather, a part of the interventionist approach to medical care.

50

Vaccinations have been linked to a number of general health problems. It now seems possible, for example, that individuals who receive vaccinations may be more prone to develop diabetes, allergies (such as asthma), arthritis, eczema and bowel disease (such as Irritable Bowel Syndrome). The explanation — which makes sense to me — is that vaccinations interfere with the immune system and make the recipients more susceptible to disease.

Who (other than a drug company spokesman) wouldn't expect an infant to show serious signs of distress when deliberately injected with potentially toxic foreign substances? Why shouldn't such injections cause a severe immune response?

51

It has also been suggested that vaccinations may be the explanation for the mystery problem 'cot death'.

Children who die of 'cot death' tend to die at exactly the sort of age when babies are having early vaccinations. Why hasn't anyone noticed that many of the babies who die of 'cot death' often die just days after the recommended dates for childhood vaccinations?

Are so-called 'cot deaths' merely another terrible consequence of government approved vaccination programmes?

52

Around the world an increasing number of parents have been arrested and charged with injuring or killing their babies. Some of those parents are undoubtedly guilty. But many (and possibly most) are not, because in many cases the baby or young child died not because he or she was attacked by a parent who had lost control but because his or her brain was damaged by a vaccine or some other medication. Shaken Baby Syndrome (in which the brain is damaged by the vaccine) is now a very real problem in all societies where vaccines are routinely (and in some countries forcibly) administered. The damage done to the baby or child by the vaccine mimics the damage that would be done if the baby was forcefully shaken. When the police investigate the sudden death of a child, and a pathologist produces a report showing that the child died because of brain damage, the chances are high that one of the parents will be charged with murder. In America this can mean that the misinformed prosecution will call for the death penalty. Naturally, doctors and drug companies deny that vaccines can kill in this or any other way.

In cases where parents (and others) have been accused of murdering their children by shaking them, or in some other way abusing them, the real culprit may well have been a vaccine. Brain damage is a well-known possible side effect of vaccination. Brain swelling, intracranial bleeding and other symptoms of 'shaken baby syndrome' can all be produced by vaccines.

None of this is widely known — perhaps because doctors and drug companies prefer unfortunate parents to take the blame for these deaths.

53

Most doctors are unquestioning — too frightened to upset the establishment. Asking uncomfortable questions can ruin a doctor's career. And medical journalists are just as useless. Most have very little formal medical training, they don't know what to look for, they not infrequently receive payments from drug companies and they hardly ever have the courage to take on the establishment. Far too many so-called medical and health journalists are wimpy incompetents who won't print or broadcast anything which might damage their cosy relationships with the medical establishment and the international pharmaceutical industry.

54

Vaccination damage can occur weeks, months or years after a vaccination.

55

Vaccines have to be developed using living systems. They are, therefore, usually cultivated in material taken from animals — in cell cultures, in fertilised hens' eggs or in the blood of infected animals. Tissues which are used include brain tissue from rabbits, kidney tissue from dogs, rabbits and monkeys, protein from hen's or duck's eggs, blood from horses or pigs. This system can, of course, be dangerous since cell cultures may be contaminated (as was the case with the polio vaccine made with monkey tissue).

Some vaccines have been prepared using bovine serum and it now appears that during the early 1990s an unknown number of children received vaccinations which may have been prepared using material from cattle which could have been infected with Bovine Spongiform Encephalitis (BSE).

Naturally, no one knows the size of the risk that was taken at the time (though it seems that the Government was warned of the hazard). And no one is likely to know the size of any problem resulting from this for at least a decade. This is yet another piece of powerful evidence supporting those who are opposed to mass vaccination programmes.

56

Vaccines also often contain additives. Antibiotics may be added to dampen down the immune system response. And stabilisers of various lands may also be included. Every time something is added to a vaccine the chances of problems developing are increased.

57

Many vaccines contain thimerosal (which contains mercury). This means that when children are vaccinated they are injected with mercury. Mercury is one of the most toxic substances on the planet. The World Health Organisation has stated that there is no safe level of mercury in the human body.

How dangerous do vaccines have to be before people stop believing the drug companies, the medical establishment and the politicians?

58

Between 20% and 50% of individuals who are vaccinated against a disease do not develop a resistance to the disease against which they have been allegedly immunised. In other words up to half of the healthy individuals who are vaccinated (and whose health and lives are therefore put at risk) gain no benefit whatsoever from the vaccination.

59

The evidence shows that diseases said to have been conquered by vaccines were in fact often controlled by other means long before vaccines were introduced.

60

Children in developing countries (often poorly fed and forced by circumstances to drink water which is dirty) are now being vaccinated by teams of workers from rich countries. Vaccination programmes are paid for by large charitable organisations. The people who give the money, and who organise the vaccination programmes, probably think they are doing good. I have no doubt at all that they are doing far more harm than good. Those organising the mass vaccination campaigns claim they are recommending vaccination as a way of preventing illness but the money would do infinitely more good (and much less harm) if it was spent on providing food and clean drinking water.

61

When companies use tissue from a bird to make a vaccine, do they have any idea how many germs may be in that tissue? Some vaccines are made with aborted human foetal tissue. Again, who knows what diseases might be carried in that tissue? Doctors using these vaccinations are practising a form of cannibalism. If you wouldn't eat someone's dead human foetus why would you want your child to be injected with tissue from that foetus?

62

Very little ongoing research is done to find out how safe or effective vaccines are. Drug companies and politicians say that vaccines are safe and effective. And people believe them. Doctors (and others) who speak out against vaccines are ignored and their work is suppressed.

63

'If I had a child now, the last thing I would allow is vaccination. I would move out of the state if I had to. I would change the family name. I would disappear. With my family. I'm not saying it would come to that. There are ways to sidestep the system with grace, if you know how to act. There are exemptions you can declare, in every state, based on religious and/or philosophic views. But if push came to shove I would go on the move.'

A former American vaccine researcher

64

Evidence that vaccines may do more harm than good is supported by experiences with animals. Between 1968 and 1988 there were considerably more outbreaks of foot and mouth disease in countries where vaccination against foot and mouth disease was compulsory than in countries where there were no such regulations. Epidemics always started in countries where vaccination was compulsory. This experience clearly shows that the alleged advantage to the community of vaccinating individuals simply does not exist.

Similar observations were made about the hyena dog, which was in 1989 threatened with extinction. Scientists vaccinated individual animals to protect them against rabies but more than a dozen packs then died within a year — of rabies. This happened even in areas where rabies had never been seen before. When researchers tried using a non-infectious form of the pathogen (to prevent the deaths of the remaining animals) all members of seven packs of dogs disappeared. And yet the rabies vaccine is now compulsory in many parts of the world. Is it not possible that it is the vaccine which is keeping this disease alive?

65

Those who eat meat should be aware that cattle (and other animals reared for slaughter) are regularly vaccinated. The meat that is taken from those animals may, therefore, contain vaccine residues in addition to hormones, antibiotics and other drugs.

66

Tragically, many doctors seem to know very little about the vaccines they advocate. In my view, if a doctor wants to vaccinate you or a member of your family you should insist that he confirm in writing that the vaccine is both entirely safe and absolutely essential. You may notice his enthusiasm for the vaccine suddenly diminish.

67

Vaccines for children and adults are compulsory in some countries. In an increasing number of countries parents who refuse to have their children vaccinated are likely to be arrested and to have their children taken away from them. In other countries (such as the UK) doctors are given a financial bonus as a reward when they 'sell' vaccinations to a large enough proportion of their patients.

As more and more people become wary about vaccines so it is likely that more and more countries will make vaccination compulsory.

68

Do influenza ('flu) vaccines work? Are they worth having?

Well, let's put it this way: I have known hundreds of doctors in my life. As far as I'm aware I have never yet known a doctor who has had a 'flu vaccine.

69

The influenza vaccine contains: different strains of influenza viruses propagated in chicken embryos; formaldehyde (used as a preservative); polyethylene glycol (used to stimulate the immune system); gelatin (made from cows' bones) and thimerosal (which contains mercury).

The strains of influenza virus used are the available strains which the drug company and the authorities guess might be the ones which will hit in the current year. The chances are, of course, that the strains of 'flu which will spread will be quite different.

The possible side effects associated with the 'flu vaccine may include: fever, tiredness, muscle aching, headache, asthma, brain swelling Guillain-Barre syndrome, facial paralysis, damage to eye muscles, damage to the arm and shoulder muscles, bruising abdominal pain, kidney disorders, hives and anaphylaxis.

It is not known whether the 'flu vaccine can trigger cancer, infertility or other serious health problems.

70

The truth is that governments are enthusiastic about vaccination not because they want to protect your child from illness (when have governments ever cared a jot about individuals?) but because they believe that vaccinations help prevent the spread of disease within a community.

The idea is a simple one.

If enough children (or, indeed, adults) are vaccinated then the incidence of that disease will hopefully be lower. Vaccinations don't by any means provide complete protection (many children who are vaccinated still develop the diseases against which they have been vaccinated) but governments hope that they may cut down the incidence of a disease.

And the advantage to a government is obvious. If, instead of a million children being ill with measles just half a million develop the disease then the number of parents having time off work will be reduced accordingly. Vaccination programmes are favoured by governments because they ease the economic burden on the State. Vaccinations are given not to prevent death or serious injury (the diseases against which vaccines are usually given do not usually kill or seriously injure anyone other than babies who are too young to have the vaccines anyway) but to protect the community.

Child A is vaccinated to stop child B getting the disease. And to help maximise the State's income.

But it is, of course, Child A who takes all the risk.

If you're a public-spirited parent then you perhaps won't mind risking your child's health (and life) for the sake of the State.

But it would be nice if they told you all this, wouldn't it?

71

Having considered the available evidence I have come to the conclusion that parents who unquestioningly trust their government and their doctor to tell them when to have their child vaccinated (and what with) are reckless beyond forgiveness and unfit to care for a child. They would deserve to have their child taken from them if this would not mean putting their child into the hands of the government and a bunch of drug company indoctrinated doctors.

And anyone who vaccinates a child should be locked up as a child abuser.

72

If you could cure all present cancers and prevent anyone ever getting cancer again by performing an experiment on one healthy child, would you go ahead — knowing that the child would certainly die?

Would you sacrifice an innocent and perfectly healthy child for the good of the community?

Let's make it more interesting. Let's assume that the child is yours.

The dilemma is a simple one.

If you allow scientists to kill your child then no one will ever again develop cancer.

Would you allow them to kill your child?

Well, in a way that's the decision your government has already made on your behalf.

They have elected to recommend (or insist) that your child be vaccinated.

Not for your child's benefit but for the good of the community. And they didn't bother to ask you what you thought about it. Instead they lied to you — telling you that the vaccinations were for your child's benefit.

Coleman's 10th Law Of Medicine

There are no holistic healers. There are only holistic patients.

1

A truly holistic approach to staying healthy and treating illness depends upon using a wide range of possible remedies; treating the patient's signs and symptoms (rather than his test results) and combining all types of alternative and orthodox medicine.

2

There are no truly holistic practitioners around. Doctors often talk about holistic medicine. So do alternative practitioners. But most of them don't have the foggiest idea what it really means.

There is, however, nothing at all to stop you being a holistic patient. For example, if your doctor tells you that you need surgery ask him how long you have got before you need to make a decision — and then use that time to make sure that you assess all the alternative possible options.

When you are trying to choose between orthodox medicine, acupuncture, homeopathy, osteopathy or whatever, make a list of all the advantages and disadvantages of every available type of therapy — and every available practitioner. Look at the claims and the potential side effects of each therapy and ask each practitioner to tell you where you can find out more. Use books and websites to educate yourself about the possibilities, advantages and hazards. Never forget that you are unique — and that your condition requires a unique solution.

3

As a holistic patient you will have to be prepared to stand your ground against health care professionals who will regard your preference for a holistic approach as bizarre.

Many orthodox practitioners are still likely to dismiss alternative or complementary medicine out of hand. If a treatment doesn't involve drugs, surgery or radiotherapy then its quackery, according to many doctors. (Curiously, young doctors are more likely to be sceptical about alternative medicine than older ones. It seems that the drug industry has, in recent years, improved its effectiveness at increasing scepticism about non-orthodox remedies. Or maybe experience does bring wisdom.)

4

Sadly, many alternative practitioners are, in their own way, just as bigoted and prejudiced. In a chapter entitled 'What I would do if I had cancer' in my book *How To Stop Your Doctor Killing You* I recommended that readers look at all the therapeutic possibilities before initiating treatment, and that they should, whenever possible, use a pick'n'mix technique; cherry picking the very best and most suitable treatment styles.

Despite my reservations and fears about them, I included drugs, surgery and radiotherapy in my list of therapies to consider. I did so because not to have done so would have been to deny the very spirit of holistic medicine. Several advocates of alternative therapies sent me very aggressive letters, accusing me of being a traitor to alternative medicine (since I am orthodox trained and have a medical degree I thought that just a trifle unfair) and of bowing to the establishment. In fact I was advocating what I believe to be true holistic medicine: an approach which includes every possible remedy and which puts the patient first. It is the patient's needs which matter most, not the vanities and preferences of individual practitioners or advocates. If you ignore or rule out whole areas of medicine because you are prejudiced against them or (even rightly) believe that they produce side effects in some patients then you are allowing your prejudices to influence your approach and you are certainly not taking a truly holistic approach.

5

A fundamental tenet of being a holistic patient is that you should learn to listen to your body. (Your body is far wiser than you imagine it to be.) And act on what it tells you. Your body knows best.

Doctors are ignorant of (and do not take advantage of) the body's own healing powers but in nine out of ten illnesses the human body is capable of healing itself without any intervention. Indeed, in many cases intervention will either slow down the healing process, or make things much worse.

Doctors don't realise just how powerful the human body is and they frequently underestimate the healing power of the body.

6

When I was working as a general practitioner I constantly wondered why some patients recovered without pills or surgery while others, with similar signs and symptoms, needed complex treatment to help them get better (and often had to put up with severe and dangerous side effects in the process).

Slowly, I discovered things that I'd never been taught in medical school or when training as a young doctor.

I found that the human body is equipped with a whole range of mechanisms designed to help keep it healthy and fight off disease.

And the body is, I discovered, equipped with a whole range of self-healing mechanisms designed to help us recover when we fall ill — without any outside help. These self-healing mechanisms have been long forgotten. (Partly I'm afraid, because drug companies can't make money out of helping patients get better by themselves).

But the more I discovered the more excited I became. As animals have known for centuries, taking medicine isn't always the quickest or the best way to get well; fasting resting staying warm and allowing the body to heal and protect itself (by using mechanisms such as vomiting and diarrhoea to eject infective organisms) may be the best way.

I called the phenomenon 'bodypower' and sat down and wrote an outline for a book I wanted to write which would show just how remarkable the forgotten powers of the human body are, how much we underestimate them and how we can use them to keep ourselves healthy and to get well again when we fall ill.

The book I wrote, in which I described the way in which the human body can defend itself, was called *Bodypower* and was first published in 1983.

One of the points I made in that book was that when the body is infected it pushes up its own temperature in order to destroy the infecting organism. When doctors prescribe pills to bring down the fever they delay the healing process by reducing the body's ability to mend itself. Medical intervention — designed to reduce the fever — interferes with the body's own self-healing mechanisms. I am constantly finding fresh evidence proving the sense of this argument. For example, I recently read about a clinical trial involving children who were suffering with chickenpox. Children who were given fever-reducing medication took a day longer to recover than those who were given a placebo sugar pill.

Much to the astonishment of the publishers *Bodypower* became an instant, huge bestseller. Since then numerous other authors around the world have described the same phenomenon.

7

Today, I am more convinced than ever of the importance of bodypower. Once you understand how bodypower works you can easily conquer nine out of ten illnesses without seeing a doctor or spending any money.

We all need doctors, hospitals and alternative therapists sometimes, of course. But if we use our bodies' own powers to protect and heal us then we need them less often than we think we do. It's sad but I suppose hardly surprising that a medical profession which is totally dominated by the pharmaceutical industry should still not embrace the principles of bodypower with unbridled enthusiasm.

8

Human bodies are very complicated. They should come with an owner's manual.

Your body is tougher than you imagine and contains numerous techniques for helping you stay alive in an emergency.

Each part of your body has powers and strengths you hardly ever use and probably aren't aware of. Only in an emergency, when you need to run faster, jump higher or fight harder than ever before in your life do your body's abilities become clear.

Appetite control

Your body contains an 'appetite control centre' designed to make sure that you eat the sort of foods you need — in the right quantities. It is our appetite control centre which makes sure that we avoid new foods unless we are reassured that they are safe to eat And it is our appetite control centre which makes us avoid certain foods when we are ill and makes us choose other foods which our bodies know we may need. So, for example, if you have hepatitis (a liver disease) you will not want to eat fatty food because with your liver in trouble your body will not be able to deal with fatty foods.

If you listen to your body — and eat only what your body wants and in the amounts it wants — then you will never get fat.

But many of us ignore our bodies. We eat at meal times rather than when we are hungry. And we eat to cheer ourselves up or because we are bored.

The result is that we get fat.

Bones

There are 200 bones in a normal, healthy body — each one specially designed for strength and movement. The biggest bone is the femur or thigh bone. Some of the smallest are the bones in your wrist. Bone has one enormous advantage over other strong materials such as steel — it can repair itself if it is damaged.

If you break a bone your body will automatically repair the damage. But, recognising that the break must have occurred at a site of weakness, the new bone will be stronger than the one you broke.

Your bones are built and joined together so well that you can lift something that weighs more than you do.

Brain

A man's brain weighs about 1.4 kg. A woman's weighs about 1.25 kg. Packed with nerve cells the brain reaches its maximum size and potential at the age of around 20 and then slowly deteriorates as cells die off. Specific parts of the brain have specific functions. For example, the back part of your brain controls your vision while the front part governs thought and personality.

Your brain contains 1,000,000,000,000 cells. Each individual cell has 5,000 connections with neighbouring cells. And every minute of every hour of every day — even while you are asleep — those cells and connections are buzzing with information.

Messages travelling along your body's nerves bring information from every individual organ and muscle.

To ensure that the right information is recognised — and acted upon — your brain will only respond when 100 identical impulses are received. Isolated bits and pieces of unsubstantiated neural 'gossip' (which could lead to a dangerously inappropriate response) are ignored. Only trends produce action.

The brain, like the rest of the body, thrives on exercise. A brain which is fed a variety of different tasks will stay healthier than one which is unused. (But the brain, like the muscles, needs rest in order to function most effectively.)

Eyes

If a speck of grit or a small fly gets into one of your eyes then tears will be produced to wash the irritant away. In addition your eyelids will temporarily go into spasm to protect your eye from further damage.

If the foreign body in your eye could be infected then the tears your eyes produce will contain an antiseptic.

Fat

Your body stores fat to provide you with emergency energy supplies. Weight for weight fat contains more stored energy than anything else.

As an extra refinement your body stores its fat in places that will make you look as attractive as possible to members of the opposite sex. That's why women store most of their fat on their bottoms, hips and breasts.

In an emergency you can live on your body's stored fat supplies for several weeks.

Heart

The average heart beats 70 times a minute. In 70 years it will beat over 2,500 million times without a service. Your body contains eight to ten pints of blood and in a day your heart will pump these eight to ten pints around your body well over a thousand times. Whatever your age and size your heart will be roughly the same size as your fist. A man's heart will weigh slightly more than a woman's heart.

Without a good, steady flow of blood your body cannot do anything. Blood carries oxygen and food supplies and removes unwanted and potentially harmful wastes.

In an emergency your heart will beat faster — going up from around 70 beats a minute to 200 beats a minute — in order to provide your tissues with extra blood and, therefore, additional food and oxygen.

Normally, your heart pumps ten pints of blood through your arteries every minute of every day. But the amount of blood your organs and tissues need will vary from minute to minute. If you are being chased by a mugger your body will need more blood than if you are slumped in a chair watching television. In an emergency — when your organs need extra supplies — your heart can pump fifty pints of blood a minute to give your muscles extra power and strength.

Intestines
Food which enters the intestinal tract begins its journey by travelling down the oesophagus or gullet. It then passes into the stomach and duodenum, before entering the small and large intestines. Altogether the whole intestinal tract is around thirty feet long — coiled inside your abdomen. The intestines have the job of digesting and breaking down the food you eat, absorbing useful nutrients and getting rid of the waste. Intestines tend to be rather idiosyncratic and what suits one person may upset another.

Kidneys
You have two kidneys, one on each side of your spine, embedded for safety in fat. Each kidney weighs just over a quarter of a pound and both contain an amazingly complex filtration system. All the blood in your body passes through your kidneys every few minutes to have the waste substances taken out of it. If your kidneys don't work properly wastes will accumulate and will eventually produce blood poisoning. Your kidneys function best if regularly flushed through with a supply of flesh, pure water.

If you go out for the evening and drink several pints of fluid your urine will become very pale and dilute.

But if you spend a day in the sun and drink very little your urine will become darker and more concentrated.

Your kidneys have the job of regulating your body's fluids so if you drink too little your kidneys will preserve liquid. But, in addition, your kidneys also ensure that salts, electrolytes and other essential chemicals are kept well-balanced. If you sweat a great deal and lose fluids and salt your kidneys will make sure that your body retains fluid and salt.

Your body has plenty of spare kidney capacity. You could lose one and a half kidneys and still have enough kidney tissue left to survive.

Liver

Your liver weighs 2.5% of your body weight and is on your right hand side looking down, just underneath your ribs. Your liver helps produce red blood cells, manufacturers antibodies which fight infection, stores iron, vitamins and carbohydrates, produces bile which helps digest fats, and breaks down drugs and poisons into waste chemicals. All this chemical activity produces so much heat that your liver plays an important part in keeping your body warm. If you consume a lot of fat or substances containing toxins, it is your liver which has the task of breaking the substances down ready for excretion. If you persistently eat too much fat and drink too much alcohol or take too many drugs then your liver will fail earlier than it might otherwise have done.

Lungs

When we are born our lungs are small, solid and yellow. When we take our first breath our lungs expand and turn pink. If you live in the country and breathe fresh air your lungs will stay pink. But if you smoke, or live in a city, your lungs gradually become darker. Your lungs ensure that the air you breathe gets into your blood to provide your tissues with oxygen.

Your body needs oxygen to survive. Under ordinary circumstances your lungs take in just a few litres of air every minute. But in a crisis your lungs increase their capacity and can bring over 100 litres of air a minute into your body.

Your body has plenty of spare lung capacity.

Muscles
Half the average person's body weight is made up of muscles. There are over 600 muscles in a normal, healthy human body. Each one is a separate organ controlled by its own nervous system and supplied by its own blood vessels. To keep the muscles in trim they need regular exercise. But they should be rested if they are sore or painful.

Navigational System
Human beings — like birds — have an inbuilt navigational system. Your system may be rusty through disuse but it is there. You have the ability to find your way home in the dark.

Pancreas
Tucked in between your stomach and your duodenum, your pancreas produces the juices and enzymes which help digest the food you eat. Cigarettes, alcohol, caffeine and too much sugar will damage the pancreas.

9

Your body contains several automatic self-healing and defence mechanisms. If you cut yourself blood will flow for a few seconds to wash away any dirt. Then special proteins will quickly form a protective net to catch blood cells and form a clot to seal the wound. The damaged cells will release special substances into your tissues to make the area red, swollen and hot. The heat kills any infection remaining and the swelling acts as a natural splint — protecting the injured area. White cells will be brought to the injury site to swallow up any bacteria. And, finally, scar tissue will build up over the wounded site. The scar tissue will be stronger than the original, damaged area of skin.

If you lose a lot of blood you will faint. This is a deliberate technique used to ensure that your brain gets a good supply of food. When you are standing your blood has to travel upwards to reach your brain. When you faint you automatically lie down and make it easier for blood to get to your brain — your most important organ.

When you have an infection your body temperature goes up. This is no coincidence. Your temperature goes up to help kill the bugs causing the infection.

If you eat something which contains toxins or poisons or infective organisms your stomach will eject it. You will vomit. If the dangerous substance or organism gets past your stomach you will develop diarrhoea. Both vomiting and diarrhoea are vital mechanisms used to getting infections out of your body as quickly as possible.

If a sweet or peanut or piece of food goes down the 'wrong way' you will cough. Your throat will narrow so that the air coming out of your lungs is put under pressure — and the obstruction will be literally blown out of the way.

10

Skin keeps the rest of the body neatly wrapped, protecting muscles and bones from injury and the weather. It also stops everything falling into an unsightly heap on the carpet. The skin on your palms and the soles of your feet is one twentieth of an inch thick but the skin on your face is ten times thinner. Peeled and stretched the average person has enough skin to make a couple of pillowcases.

If you use your hands a lot to perform heavy, manual work you will eventually develop patches of coarse, hard skin. The patches of hard skin will develop in precisely the areas where your body needs to be toughest.

The same thing happens elsewhere.

So, if you do a lot of walking you will develop thick areas of skin on your feet. These will ensure that your skin is hard wearing in places where it needs to be hard wearing. It's like having a pair of shoes that automatically strengthen themselves in the places where they look likely to wear out.

In addition your skin also has an inbuilt mechanism designed to stop you getting sunburnt.

If you spend a lot of time in the sun special cells will release a substance called melanin which slowly turns your skin brown and provides protection against damage. Dark skinned people — who come from sunny countries — are born with a protective layer of melanin in their skins.

In hot or windy weather skin tends to dry out and crack. This is a particular problem in air-conditioned buildings where the air is often dry. To keep skin in good condition it needs regular moisturising with a plain cream.

11

Your body can survive only if its internal temperature remains within a narrow temperature range — above 30 degrees C and below 45 degrees C.

So how do you survive when the outside temperature is lower or higher than these limits?

Easy.

Your body contains a thermostat which maintains a stable internal temperature. When the outside temperature is too hot you lose heat through sweat. And when the outside temperature is too low you automatically shiver to keep yourself warm.

12

The human body has enormous, hidden strengths and far greater power than most of us ever realise.

We tend to think of ourselves as being delicate and vulnerable. But our bodies are tougher than we imagine, far more capable of coping with physical and mental stresses and far better equipped for self-defence. As proof of this there is, for example, the true story of the nine stone mother who lifted three quarters of a ton of motorcar off her nine-year-old son, Jamie.

Few of us fulfil our physical (or mental) potential or succeed in harnessing the powers we have available within us. Very few of us know the extent of own strength. Only if we are pushed to our limits do we find out precisely what we can do.

The story of the nine stone woman who lifted her three quarters of a ton car off her young son is not unique.

I know of at least three other cases where parents have done exactly the same thing.

Here are some other examples of human beings finding superhuman powers.

* A zoologist working in Africa was being chased by wild animals in the dark. He leapt up into a tree. The following morning, at dawn, he discovered that he

had leapt twelve feet into the air. When he finally got down from the tree he could not even reach the branch he'd leapt onto.

* A 70-year-old Irish farmer woke to find his home on fire. He climbed onto the roof and walked along a telegraph wire 9 yards along. Then he climbed down the telegraph pole to the ground. He had never walked a tightrope in his life.

* During the Second World War a special agent on a ship that was being attacked by a German submarine dragged a safe onto deck ready to throw it overboard. When the attack was over — it took four men to carry the safe back down again.

* A farm labourer whose arm had been chopped off in an accident walked several miles to the nearest hospital — carrying his severed arm!

* An 87-year-old widow, trapped in her bedroom by a fire, knotted sheets together and climbed down them to safety.

13

In an emergency your body makes a number of preparations to help you cope. In effect, when you are in danger your body responds as though a soldier reacting to the command Battle Stations.

* Your pupils dilate so that your vision becomes more acute.

* Your hearing becomes sharper. (Animals prick up their ears but humans have lost this skill).

* When you're trying to listen for important sounds — or see things that might help save your life — your heartbeat will temporarily slow down and your breathing will stop for a moment or two to help you look and listen for vital clues.

* The flow of blood to your brain increases so that you can make decisions more rapidly than ever.

* The flow of blood to your skin is reduced (and you go pale). This means that if you're injured your blood loss will be kept to a minimum.

* Acid will flow into your stomach to ensure that any food there is turned into sugar rapidly — to provide you with energy.

* Your muscles will be tensed — so that you can run or fight.

* Your breathing rate will go up so that your lungs bring in plenty of oxygen.

* Your heart rate will go up so that the supply of blood to your organs increases.

14

You know your own body better than anyone. If you feel that there is something wrong then there is probably something wrong.

15

You are particularly unlikely to find a holistic specialist.

If you visit a Ford dealer he will want to sell you a Ford. Not a BMW. Not a bicycle. Not a pair of roller skates. A Ford. And if you visit an Ear Nose and Throat surgeon he will want to look down your throat. If you complain of bunions to an ENT surgeon he will still want to look down your throat.

If you visit a surgeon the chances are that he will want to operate. Visit a physician with the same symptoms and he will probably want to give you pills. Surgeons operate and physicians hand out pills. And ENT surgeons look down throats. It's what they do. Doctors think in the boxes into which they have put themselves.

So, too, do alternative practitioners.

Visit an acupuncturist and he will stick needles into you. Visit a herbalist and he will give you herbs to take. Very few herbalists will recommend acupuncture and vice versa.

16

If your health problem isn't an emergency, you should always study all the options before you accept treatment.

17

Don't assume that your doctor knows as much as you or he thinks he knows (or would like to think he knows).

18

Practitioners of oriental medicine in general, and Chinese medicine in particular, tend to strive to treat every infection in a holistic way. If a patient has an infection, for example, they will assume that the pathogen is not the direct and sole cause of the disease but that its ability to infect the body is merely a symptom of some internal imbalance; a consequence of a disrupted physiological or psychological homeostasis.

If the infection is to be treated properly then the underlying imbalance must also be put right. Simply attacking the pathogen will provide only a short-term solution.

In modern, orthodox medicine western doctors treat infectious diseases by attacking the pathogen which they believe to be responsible. They do not consider that there may be other factors involved. They do not consider that an infection might have taken hold because the body was weakened in some way and they do not realise that attacking only the bug is effectively treating a symptom rather than a cause.

In fact it isn't only Chinese practitioners who take this holistic approach. Animals do it too. They know that they are more susceptible to infection during times of drought, famine and overcrowding when their bodies are under stress. Their response to infection is far more sensible than our own.

19

Although they do learn from one another, and will often help a sick relative or companion, animals don't rely on outside help when they are ill; they self-medicate. Their aim, of course is to re-establish a feeling of well-being. In order to do this they must understand their own bodies.

20

The animals on modern farms are denied the opportunity to treat themselves. They are crammed into fields or barns where there is little space and little or no opportunity to self-medicate by changing their diet. All they have available to eat is what is provided by the farmer: grass (if they are in a field) or special feed mixture (if they are in a barn). Their diet bears no relationship to the sort of food they would choose to eat. Farmers feed animal waste to vegetarian animals. In the USA farmers feed chicken excrement directly to cattle, to give them protein. In addition to this American farmers feed cattle and pigs: human sewage, dead cats and dogs, slaughterhouse waste (blood, bones, intestines and their contents), cement kiln dust, old newspapers, waste cardboard, agricultural waste and old fat from restaurants and grease traps. In France farmers feed human sewage to French cattle. Mad Cow Disease developed in Britain because farmers fed cattle the ground up brains and spinal cords of other animals. Those who eat meat are, of course, eating parts of animals fed on this horrendously unhealthy diet. If farmers knew anything about their animals they would know that herbivorous ruminants don't eat meat and never, ever engage in cannibalism.

The animals on modern farms are often denied sunlight and exercise. The farmer's sole aim is to turn the animal into meat (and other products) and eventually into profit. There is no access to the variety of natural plants which enable them to self-medicate. The result of the physical overcrowding is that parasites and disease spread quickly and easily, psychological problems develop and the animals cannot treat themselves. The treatment comes from the farmer and, inevitably, involves the use of powerful drugs. Often drugs such as antibiotics are included in the animal's feed on a long-term basis. When an animal falls ill it is in the farmer's commercial interest to hide or cover up any illness if there is a chance that this may restrict the farmer's ability to add the animal to the food chain. The piece of meat you buy from the butcher or supermarket could contain a hidden lump of cancer.

21

When animals are ill they take a holistic approach to self-healing. If, for example, they have an infection they will take a variety of different types of action to protect and mend themselves. So, for example, if they have intestinal parasites, chimps will do three things: they will chew plants which contain multifunctional healing compounds; they will eat termite mound soil which is able to secrete antibodies and which has the medicinal healing properties of clay (see item 24 in this chapter) and they will swallow up folded hairy leaves which catch worms and help speed their expulsion.

22

When allowed to live naturally, chickens live in small groups in woodland areas. They scratch around on the forest floor eating worms, insects and bits of fresh plant. They use the dust and the sunshine to keep their feathers bright and when it rains they take a shower to add a little lustre. At night they roost in trees (their claws are adapted for hanging onto branches even while they are asleep) so that they are safe from predators.

Chicken farmers have selectively bred chickens to grow faster and faster. They have doubled the maturing speed in the last two decades and have created birds who grow so fast that their heart and circulation cannot cope. The birds are constantly ill. Their bones are incapable of supporting their excess weight and so they frequently suffer broken bones. They then die of thirst and starvation because they cannot reach the automated food and water delivery points in their cages.

Eight out of ten broiler chickens suffer broken bones. Around 17,0000 birds a day die in the UK of heart failure. The chicken farmers regard this as an affordable cost. The food the chickens are given is selected according to price. One of the ingredients is ground up dead chickens. The chickens are routinely fed antibiotics (to stop the weakened birds getting infections and to help boost muscle growth) despite the danger that this creates for humans. They are kept in the half dark so that they keep quiet and there is, of course, no air- conditioning so in hot weather the heat in their cages is unbearable. The chickens stand in their own excrement (which is acidic and so it blisters their feet) and they breathe in fumes; dust and bacteria from their neighbours. They are given no freedom and no chance to self medicate. Despite the fact that many broiler flocks are colonised with bugs which can cause neurological problems, arthritis, headache, backache, fever, nausea, pains and diarrhoea millions of people eat chicken every day.

23

Doctors and scientists experiment on animals in a vain attempt to find new cures for human ailments and yet they learn little or nothing from observing animals. Holistic practitioners should learn from everything they see or hear.

24

From animals we can (or should) learn that successful good health depends primarily on avoidance and prevention. Treatment is a last resort — to be used when things have gone wrong.

Doctors haven't learned much from animals because neither avoiding illness nor preventing it offer great opportunities for profit.

Doctors could learn a great deal too by watching how animals deal with disease. For example, cattle will treat themselves when they are ill if they are given the chance (which they usually aren't).

Ranchers in Utah used to turn out sick cattle who had diarrhoea, expecting them to fend for themselves in the wild. They were surprised when, after a few days away the cattle returned, quite well again. What had happened was that the cattle had travelled to clay banks and had fed on the clay until they got better again. Clay works very effectively in the treatment of intestinal poisoning because it absorbs toxins and viruses. In the UK the medicinal benefits of clay are ignored and so every year 170,000 calves die of diarrhoea caused by bacterial infections. (This only goes to prove how stupid the average farmer must be. How much does clay cost?)

Cattle aren't the only animals to use clay to counteract the effects of poisoning. Animals throughout the world use clay for this purpose, knowing that it detoxifies by binding onto harmful substances. Why don't humans use clay? Why don't doctors prescribe it? Why don't first aid kits contain clay pills? The answer, as it so often is, is bureaucracy. In the UK, for example, foods and medicines are dealt with by different Government departments and clay isn't accepted as a food or a medicine. So it can't be prescribed or used by anyone except wild animals.

Coleman's 11th Law Of Medicine

There is no such thing as minor surgery.

1

Some operations are more complicated than others. Some take longer to perform. Some are more dangerous. All surgery should be taken seriously. It is never safe to describe surgery as 'minor'.

Coleman's 12th Law Of Medicine

Some patients will always be treated more equally than others.

1

Today it is the elderly who are treated least equally.

2

When I was a medical student I was a member of a well-meaning organisation called, I think, the Medical Association for the Prevention of War. At a conference I attended I remember being shocked to the core to discover that one doctor had observed that, in riots in one American city, hospitals had given precedence to the treatment of injured police officers to the detriment of seriously injured demonstrators. Incoming patients were not treated according to their need, but according to the clothes they wore.

Sadly, it seems that wherever there is a hospital there will be prejudice.

Apart from obvious geographical inequalities (patients in some areas receive far better care than patients in more poorly served areas) there are many examples showing that even on a national scale health care is not distributed fairly or evenly among those who need it. The problem is that politicians, administrators and doctors invariably spend money on those who are perceived to have power. Those who are regarded as powerless may be denied even basic care. So, for example, while infertility treatment is widely offered to those who need it governments happily close down long-stay psychiatric care hospitals without providing any alternative. Community care means that long-stay hospitals are closed and the homeless patients discharged to spend their days and nights in bus shelters and amid the rat infested squalor underneath city flyovers. That's what 'care in the community' means. Those who are able and willing to promote their own needs (either in the media or directly to politicians) will always receive more than those who are not so fortunate. This is particularly true wherever socialist medicine is practised. In Britain the constantly ailing National Health Service, ostensibly designed to provide equal care for all, is grotesquely biased towards the photogenic and towards those noisy and demanding liberals who can make sure that their demands are met at the expense of the rest of the community. The mentally ill, not as good at arguing their case as those young media women demanding yet more resources for breast cancer, get forgotten. Celebrities will wear pink ribbons to remind us of the needs of breast cancer patients but how many would proclaim their interest in bowel cancer — a much bigger killer? Making a decision between closing a breast cancer unit or closing a special needs school won't tax a politician for long.

3

These days there is no doubt that the patients who are treated with least respect are the elderly. They get an even worse deal than the mentally ill — and that, believe me, is saying a lot.

In the summer of 2006, for example, newspapers carried the appalling story of a 91-year-old woman who spent her last four days without food or fluids after hospital staff decided not to provide her with either. When the woman asked a nurse for a cup of tea she was told she couldn't have one. The woman's family obtained a High Court injunction to try to force the hospital to treat the woman. But, nevertheless, a pathologist concluded that the woman had died as a result of lack of food and fluids.

Such stories are increasingly commonplace.

The egregious doctors who behave like this are simply doing what their Government wants them to do. To ruthless politicians the elderly are a drain on society; they have to be paid pensions, they use up expensive medical services and they pay very little in the way of taxes.

4

It is traditional, in mammalian species, for wisdom to be passed from generation to generation. The elderly have much to offer to the younger generation. In return for this knowledge, and in respect, the young care for their elders with care, compassion and consideration.

So, for example, the situation of underground water sources will be remembered by older elephants. This knowledge can save the herd during a drought. Younger elephants are so aware of the value of their elders, and so in awe of them, that when older elephants are slaughtered by poachers the young, orphaned elephants suffer from severe behavioural problems. They fail to find enough food for themselves, they don't know what to do or where to go and they end up running amok, killing farmers and raiding their crops. They fight one another. They become yobs. Without access to their elders the young elephants are doomed to conflict.

Much the same thing happens with lions.

Young lions recognise that older lions can help with the complex cooperative hunting strategies which lions me to catch their prey. And so older lionesses, incapable of hunting and, became of missing teeth doomed to die if not cared for, will live out their old age supported by the younger females.

Chimpanzees care for their elderly too. Elderly chimpanzees are given food and groomed by the other members of their society. Older male chimpanzees aren't subjected to the sort of aggression other males must expect, and their own rather feeble aggressive behaviour will be tolerated without retaliation by younger males.

Old age brings respect in much of the animal world. But not for humans.

In our modern society we pay respect only to youth, technology (whether useful or not), money (however acquired) and fame (whether deserved or not). The abuse of the elderly is ignored, even tolerated, in a way that the abuse of children would never be.

5
'Old age is not for cissies.'

Bette Davis

6
More older people die during winter in the UK than in any other European country — including those countries which are colder. This is due to poor housings poor diet, poverty, not enough state support, neglect, depression caused by loneliness, and a general feeling of being unwanted and uncared for.

7
The system wants you dead as soon as you stop working and paying tax. And the system now decides what happens. People don't control the system.

8
In America in April 2006 an 82-year-old woman was arrested and fined £80 for crossing the road too slowly in Los Angeles. She was walking with a cane and just

couldn't get across the road before the lights turned red.

I do hope they remembered to give the policemen an award for bravery.

9

There are around 600 million people in the world aged 60 or over. But this will double by 2025 and reach 2,000 million by 2050.

10

'The doctors told me that my mother was dying,' wrote a reader. 'They convinced me and my brother that they should shut off her ventilator and let her die. But a few minutes after they had shut off the ventilator my mother woke up and wanted to know what was for tea. She danced at her 89th birthday party the following week.'

I have great sympathy for the writer of that letter. My own mother was written off by the teaching hospital where she was a patient early in a long illness in her 80's. She was comatose and although they admitted that they didn't know what was wrong with her, they decided that she was terminally ill and should be left to die. Only our insistence that they keep providing her with fluids via an intravenous drip kept her alive. Who, I wondered aloud, gave doctors, nurses and administrators the right to make this sort of judgement?

Eighteen months later my mother had recovered enough to join my father, myself and my wife at a dinner to celebrate their 65th wedding anniversary. I photographed her with a glass of red wine in her hand and a big smile on her face. Curiously none of the doctors who had described her as terminally ill, and who had abandoned her as beyond care, has shown any interest in her astonishing recovery.

11

Ageism is accepted now in our society. It is the only 'ism' which is deemed to be politically acceptable.

12

After leaving the teaching hospital my mother was in a small cottage hospital which wanted to throw her out. They said they wanted the bed for another patient. My mother was incapable of moving any limb. She could do nothing for herself. She was so confused that she didn't recognise me when I visited.

'We've got a shortage of beds,' said the matron. 'Your mother will have to go home.' She told me that I had to attend a meeting.

The meeting was held in a fully-equipped but entirely empty ward.

No one but me saw the irony in this.

13

I have often wondered why doctors seem to hate old people so much.

In the end I came to the conclusion that it is because they cannot stop them dying.

And the death of a patient is, to a doctor, the ultimate insult; the final sign of professional failure.

14

Both the Government and the medical profession have repeatedly announced that old people will, on occasion, be denied normal medical treatment and will be allowed to die.

It is now standard practice for elderly patients (in some hospitals the cut off point may be as low as 60 or

65) to be denied medical help if they need resuscitation or emergency, life-saving treatment. In some hospitals the elderly are deliberately starved to death so that they don't take up valuable beds for too long.

Old people are treated in a way that would not be tolerated if they were members of a religious group or ethnic group.

For example, in the paragraphs above try replacing the word 'elderly' with the word 'Jews'.

I can't see any Government happily encouraging newspapers to run headlines like: 'Politicians Instruct Hospitals To Let Jews Die'.

15

Now that nurses have been given authority to prescribe drugs even more old people are spending their final years in a drug-induced stupor.

In hospitals and nursing homes everywhere elderly patients are being subdued and sedated with tranquillisers and sleeping tablets.

It's much easier to run either type of institution if the inmates spend most of their time sleeping.

Politicians have made things considerably worse by giving nurses legal authority to give old people drugs without their permission or authorisation.

The result of this is that hundreds of thousands of elderly people spend their final years unaware of what is going on around them; forcibly drugged into State-approved senselessness.

Makes you ashamed to be human doesn't it?

16

A friend of mine who is a doctor tells me that every time he visits his mother (who now resides in an expensive nursing home) he finds her asleep. Each time he visits he demands to see the drug records. He finds

out that his mother has been drugged and insists that
the medication be withdrawn. For a few days his
mother becomes alert and awake. Then, when they get
fed up of her asking to be given a cup of tea or taken to
the toilet, the staff start sedating her again.

17

My mother was still lying in a hospital bed. She had
been (wrongly) diagnosed as suffering from terminal
cancer. She had been in a coma for several weeks and
had only recently woken up and started to take an
interest in her surroundings. She was still unable to
move or feed herself. She had a catheter fitted and was
being nursed on a special vibrating bed because of
bedsores. Despite the diagnosis and her physical
condition the hospital once again decided to discharge
her from hospital in order to free a bed and save
money. I was again summoned to a meeting. This time
there were nine (nine) health service employees
present. There was one doctor, one nurse and seven
people whose jobs I didn't quite catch. They looked
like administrators. Seven of them. I suspect that the
cost of the meeting (and the preparations for it) would
have paid for quite a few patients lives to be saved.

'According to the hospital consultant my mother is
terminally ill with cancer,' I reminded them.

'Yes,' said one of the administrators. 'But she's not
finally terminally ill.'

The emphasis was on the word 'finally'. I swear the
administrator smiled as he delivered what he clearly
considered to be a clever coup de grace.

As it happens the diagnosis was wrong.

But what sort of administrator invented the phrase
'not finally terminally ill' as an excuse for throwing a
sick patient out of hospital?

18

If old people have money and can afford to pay for their own nursing home care they will be discharged and expected to spend their resources paying for their own care.

If they don't have money they will simply be sent home to look after themselves as well as they can.

Two social workers/bureaucrats/inquisitors were questioning a frail old lady in a hospital bed. The woman was clearly confused and demented. The two inquisitors had been sent to question her to assess her fitness to be sent back home. I happened to be in the hospital visiting a friend. I listened to their questioning and wrote down their questions and the answers immediately afterwards.

'You have a son don't you?' said the first inquisitor, the one holding the clipboard.

The old lady looked puzzled.

'You have a son.'

'Thank you.'

'What does he do for a living?'

'Living?'

'What's his job?'

The old lady thought for a while. 'Teacher,' she said.

The inquisitor nodded patronisingly. 'Splendid,' she said. Without making any attempt to find out whether or not the answer was correct she wrote something on the form she was filling in.

The inquisitor then asked the old lady what her husband had done for a living before he retired.

The old lady clearly didn't know.

'He was a teacher,' she said.

'Do you have a fridge at home?' asked the inquisitor.

The old woman looked bewildered.

'A fridge,' repeated the inquisitor rather impatiently.

'What's that?' asked the old lady, looking very confused.

'A big white thing that keeps food cold.'

'I don't know.'

'I'm sure you have,' said the inquisitor. She turned to her companion. 'She'll have a fridge won't she?'

'Oh I expect so,' nodded the companion, though the old lady clearly didn't know what a fridge was, let alone whether or not she had one.

'We will put you down as having one,' the inquisitor said, as though doing her a favour. 'It's good for keeping frozen food.'

The inquisitor with the clipboard ticked a box. The two inquisitors then signed the form and stood up.

They had officially declared that the old lady was neither confused nor demented.

'Why didn't you just chuck her out of the window?' I thought. It would be quicker for everyone and just as kindly.

Twenty minutes after the inquisitors had left the woman's son arrived. When he had found a vase for the flowers he had brought he sat down by his mother's bedside.

I went over to him, apologised for interrupting and asked if I might have a moment of his time.

He stood up and walked with me into the dayroom. I told him about the visit I'd witnessed.

'They want to send my mum home,' said the man. 'She's 82 and lives alone in a terraced house. They said they'd assess her to see if she's capable of looking after herself.'

'Can I ask you if you're a teacher?' I asked.

He laughed. 'A teacher? Me?' He laughed again. 'Who told you that?'

'Your mother told the inquisitors that you're a teacher.'

'She gets confused,' said the man. 'Most of the time she doesn't even know who I am. I'm a car mechanic.'

'Is your father a teacher?'

'Did she say that?'

I nodded.

He shook his head sadly. There was a tear in the corner of one eye. 'They were married for nearly 60 years,' he told me. 'He was a taxi driver. He died eighteen months ago.'

'They're going to send your mother home,' I told him quietly. 'They think she's capable of looking after herself.'

'She's doubly incontinent, she's diabetic and she doesn't recognise anyone,' said the man, quietly desperate. 'My wife and I live in a one bedroom flat. We can't look after her. They can't send her home.' But they could. And they did.

19

My novel *Mrs Caldicot's Cabbage War* describes the revolt of a pensioner, dumped in a nursing home by her son and daughter-in-law. Mrs Caldicot can't stand the way she is patronised by the proprietor of the home. And she can't stand the smell of cabbage either. She walks out — and the other residents go with her. The book describes what happens. When the movie of the book was released the reviewer in the *Sunday Times* dismissively and patronisingly described the film's target audience as 'undemanding oldies'. I though it ironic that a book and film written to draw attention to rampant ageism should be the subject of such rampant ageism. I wonder if a critic would have dared describe a film about homosexuals as having been made for 'undemanding poofs'? I suspect not.

20

My wife and I decided to take my parents out for a meal to celebrate a birthday. Both were aged 85 at the time and both could only get about in wheelchairs.

We made arrangements for a local taxi firm to send a special taxi capable of carrying a passenger in a wheelchair.

Instead the taxi firm sent an ordinary taxi which was, of course, quite useless. The driver couldn't care less.

We decided we would wheel my parents to the nearest hotel or pub for lunch. But the only place that was open had no access for wheelchairs.

So, in desperation, we wheeled them to a local chip shop for a bag of chips each. Although my parents are resident in a nursing home in a seaside town which is packed with nursing homes and elderly residents we discovered that the kerbs had not been made wheelchair friendly. So we had to bump both chairs up and down countless steep kerbs.

By this time it was, of course, raining heavily.

Since there was no wheelchair access to the chip shop we ate our bags of chips on the pavement in the rain.

As we did so a group of local youths passed by. They laughed and jeered.

21

The more vulnerable a patient is, and the more he or she needs care, the less he or she is likely to receive it. Especially if he or she is elderly.

22

My wife and I were visiting a friend at a nursing home. As we approached the main building we saw an old man stumble and fall. We made sure that he was not injured and then struggled to help him to his feet. Two employees (hired to care for the elderly people living in the nursing home) stood looking out of a window and laughing at our struggles.

23

The official guidelines for doctors are simple and easy to understand. 'Doctors,' they say, 'must not allow their views about, for example, a patient's age, disability, race, colour, culture, beliefs, sexuality, gender, lifestyle, social or economic status to prejudice the choices of treatment offered or the general standard care provided. Patients who are dying should be afforded the same respect and standard of care as all other patients.'

It is clear from this, when compared to my own experience and that of many of my readers, than the majority of hospital doctors are in breach of these principles and are unfit to practise.

24

At the end of the day most doctors and nurses don't give a damn whether you live or die. And if you're over 65 everyone wants you dead. Remember that. It could save your life one day.

The Author

Instinctively anti-authority and recklessly uncompromising, Vernon Coleman is the iconoclastic author of well over 100 books which have sold over 2 million copies in the UK, been translated into 23 languages and now sell in over 50 countries. His best-selling nonfiction book *Bodypower* was voted one of the 100 most popular books of the 1980s/90s and was turned into two television series in the UK. The film of his novel *Mrs Caldicot's Cabbage War* was released early in 2003. In the 1980s, although several of his books had been high in the bestseller lists, he got fed up with nervous publishers trying to edit all the good bits out of his books and so he started his own publishing conglomerate which began life in a barn and now employs five people.

Vernon Coleman has written columns for the *Daily Star, Sun, Sunday Express, Planet on Sunday* and *The People* (resigning from the latter when the editor refused to publish a column questioning the morality and legality of invading Iraq) and has contributed over 5,000 articles, columns and reviews to 100 leading British publications including *Daily Telegraph, Sunday Telegraph, Guardian, Observer, Sunday Times, Daily Mail, Mail on Sunday, Daily Express, Woman, Woman's Own, Punch* and *Spectator*. His columns and articles have also appeared in hundreds of leading magazines and newspapers throughout the rest of the world. He edited the *British Clinical Journal* for one year until a drug company told the publisher to choose between firing him or getting no more advertising. For twenty years he wrote a column which was syndicated to over 40 leading regional newspapers. Eventually, the column had to be abandoned when Government-hired doctors offered to write alternative columns without charge to stop him telling readers the truth. His first two books on medicine *(The Medicine Men* and *Paper Doctors)* were well and widely reviewed, though they attracted a good deal of petulant criticism from magazines which existed upon drug company advertising and from members of the medical establishment His subsequent books on similar topics (such as *The Health Scandal, Betrayal of Trust* and *How to Stop Your Doctor Killing You)* were ignored by the media, even though they sold much better and attracted far more interest from readers. Over the years many attempts have been made to suppress his books. In the UK advertisements for *How To Stop Your Doctor Killing You* were quite simply banned. It was allegedly feared that the title might upset doctors.

In the UK Vernon Coleman was the TV AM doctor on breakfast TV and when he commented that fatty food had killed more people than Hitler he wasn't fired until several weeks after a large food lobbyist had threatened to pull all its advertising. He was the first networked television Agony Aunt. In the past he has presented TV and radio programmes for both BBC and commercial channels though these days no producer who wants to keep his job for long is likely to invite him anywhere near a studio (especially a BBC studio). Many millions consulted his Telephone Doctor advice lines and visited his websites and for six years he wrote a monthly newsletter which had subscribers in 17 countries. Vernon Coleman has a medical degree, and an honorary science doctorate. He has worked for the Open University in the UK and is an honorary Professor of Holistic Medical Sciences at the Open International University based in Sri Lanka. He used to give occasional lectures but these days the invitations are usually withdrawn when big companies find out about it.

Vernon Coleman has received lots of really interesting awards from people he likes and respects. He is, for example, a Knight Commander of The Ecumenical Royal Medical Humanitarian Order of Saint John of Jerusalem, of the Knights of Malta and a member of the Ancient Royal Order of Physicians dedicated to His Majesty King Buddhadasa. In 2000 he was awarded the Yellow Emperor's Certificate of Excellence as Physician of the Millennium by the Medical Altemativa Institute. He is also Vice Chancellor of the Open International University. He has not been offered, and would not accept, any award by the British Government.

He has had an interest in medicine for most of his life (having bought and read the Royal College of Physicians Report on smoking with his pocket money when he was ten years old). He worked as a general practitioner for ten years (resigning from the NHS after being fined for refusing to divulge confidential information about his patients to State bureaucrats) and has organised numerous campaigns both for people and for animals. He is enraged by injustice, inhumanity and oppressive authority and relieves his rage by collecting hobbies and accumulating books (though buying books faster than anyone could possibly read them creates problems too). He has been intending to learn to speak French for over half a century but has made very little progress. He can ride a bicycle and swim, though not at the same time. He is delighted to report that he researched and wrote this book without the aid of Microsoft, Windows or any of their contemporaries, and consequently estimates that he did it in half the time it would otherwise have taken. He loves cats, cricket (before they started painting slogans on the grass), cycling, cafés and, most of all, the Welsh Princess.

Vernon Coleman is balding rapidly and is widely disliked by members of the Establishment. He doesn't give a toss about either of these facts. Many attempts have been made to ban his books but he insists he will keep writing them even if he has to write them out in longhand and sell them on street corners (though he hopes it doesn't come to this because he still has a doctor's handwriting). He is married to Donna Antoinette, the totally adorable Welsh Princess, and is very pleased about this. Together they have written two books *How To Conquer Health Problems Between Ages 50 And 120* and *Health Secrets Doctors Share With Their Families.*

An Interview with Dr Vernon Coleman

This interview is a composite, consisting of frequently asked questions, and is based on interviews conducted on behalf of magazines in different parts of the world. The interview concentrates on Vernon Coleman's work as a medical author.

Q: Are you a medically qualified doctor? What provoked your scepticism about the medical profession?

A: I am a qualified doctor and registered to practice — though I have not done so for many years. Doctors are necessary and do much good. But my scepticism is, I fear, based on sound scientific basis and my criticisms largely concern the way the medical establishment is organised and the way doctors have allowed themselves to be influenced by commercial forces. I have researched what doctors do with a critical eye and I have proved that too often doctors do more harm than good. In many countries doctors are now one of the three or four main causes of illness and death (along with cancer and circulatory disease). One in six patients in hospital is there because he or she has been made ill by doctors. Four out of ten patients who receive drug treatment suffer from serious or even life-threatening side effects. It is perhaps hardly surprising that when doctors go on strike, patient morbidity and mortality levels invariably fall. What an indictment.

Q: Do you take medicines if you are ill? If not how do to make yourself well if you fall ill?

A: I will take medicines if I need them and believe that the advantages outweigh the disadvantages. But most problems can be dealt with without drugs.

Q: Do you think that doctors are influenced too much by the pharmaceutical industry?

A: I have been a strong critic of the relationship between the pharmaceutical industry and the medical profession since 1976 when I published my first book *The Medicine Men* in which I described the way that the industry influences and controls the medical profession. It is easy to blame the drug industry (and many of their practices do seem to me to be grotesquely unethical) but I do think that the medical profession should take more of the blame. The drug companies are doing what they are in business to do — make money. It should be up to doctors to be more critical. I don't feel that much has changed over the last thirty years (since I first started writing books on this subject) and the drug companies still have an enormous control over doctors and what they believe. The industry still has enormous influence over all aspects of medical education, and doctors are trained to believe that the only answer to medical problems is, very often, some form of pharmaceutical intervention. That is wrong and it is dangerous.

Q: Surely; medicines must sometimes be used to cure Illness.

A: Definitely. I am certainly not opposed to the use of medicines but I am opposed to their overuse and abuse. For example, the overprescribing of antibiotics has led to enormous problems — including the development of superbugs. I have been warning about this problem for decades and forecast the emergence of superbugs some decades ago. The overuse of tranquillisers led to the biggest addiction problem of the 20th century. And often doctors don't really know what they are prescribing or why. For example, doctors sometimes prescribe antibiotics for viral infections (a pointless exercise) and while some doctors give out prescriptions of antibiotics for ten days others give five or even three day courses for the same symptoms. Ignorance and illogically cause many problems. In the area of painkillers doctors are often too free to use pills when in many instances other methods would be safer and more effective. For example, TENS machines are very effective for combating pain but many doctors don't know about them. The drug industry and the medical establishment have conspired to keep them secret.

Q: More and more people are now turning to traditional, complementary or alternative medicine. Do you believe that more doctors are now convinced of the usefulness of these types of medicine?
A: Sadly, doctors are, as a group, still reluctant to accept that alternative medicine can offer patients a great deal. Occasionally, doctors attend a weekend course in, say, acupuncture, and then believe that they are holistic practitioners. Holistic medicine means treating the patients with whatever is best for him or her and this is only rarely seen. Sadly, some alternative therapists are so opposed to orthodox medicine that they too fail their patients. In an ideal world the patient would be treated with whatever therapies work best — and with whatever combination of therapies are most effective. It is a tragedy that this is so rare.

Q: Are doctors who prescribe alternative treatments behaving responsibly?
A: Yes. Definitely. As long as they have studied the treatments they recommend. For example, a good doctor should always consider referring patients with back or joint trouble to an osteopath or chiropractor rather than just to a surgeon. I strongly believe in holistic medicine; by which I mean that doctors should

prescribe whatever might help a patient get well again. In the absence of holistic practitioners' patients should aspire to be holistic patients.

Q: How can the patient learn the balance between orthodox and alternative medicine?
A: Every patient needs to be their own doctor — able to take a real part in the diagnosing and treatment of conditions. Books are still by far the best way to acquire information.

Q: Do you suspect that doctors ever have any personal interest in recommending medicines from specific companies?
A: There is much evidence showing that doctors can be 'bought' with free meals, television sets and other gifts. Their prescribing habits can be influenced by drug company representatives.

Q; Surely researchers wouldn't have the funds to find new drugs to cure diseases if they were not paid by the drug companies?
A We need a pharmaceutical industry. It would be good if the industry was more honest but I think we should blame doctors for that. Doctors should keep drug companies more honest by being more critical. And doctors should be more independent and should realise that drugs are only part of what they can do for patients. Unfortunately, there is evidence to show that drug companies influence the medical establishment and the medical way of thinking with the result that patients lose out. It is also important to remember that much drug company research goes into developing what are called 'me too' drugs — where the company involved simply wants to produce another drug to take advantage of an existing market. And it is for this reason that there are a hundred different painkillers —

all doing much the same thing — for doctors to choose from. Too much choice can sometimes be bad because it causes confusion and mistakes. Incidentally, the overall influence of the drug companies on our health has been dramatically over emphasised. The main influences on our health come from food, water, living and working conditions and so on. The figures show that mortality rates have not improved in the last century. Infant mortality rates have fallen a great deal because of better housing, better water and so on and these improvements have affected overall life expectancy figures. But drug companies (and doctors) like to pretend that we are all living longer because of drugs. This simply isn't true.

Q: Are you opposed to the use of anti-depressants? Do you think that depression is a disease created by the drug industry?
A: When my campaign against the overprescribing of tranquillisers led directly to a fall in the number of prescriptions I forecast that drug companies would start pushing anti-depressants much harder. This is exactly what they did. Anti-depressants are now often prescribed for people who are unhappy or who have lifestyle problems. The overprescribing of these drugs in unsuitable circumstances causes many additional problems.

Q: What other diseases do you think are also 'created' by the medical industry?
A: It is frequently claimed that asthma is much commoner than it was. But in fact these days doctors diagnose asthma after a child wheezes just once. And then the patient may be put on drugs for life. Few doctors take the time to look for causes. Many chemicals in the home (for example, soap powder) can

cause wheezing. Remove the cause and the problem disappears. And many doctors prescribe antihypertensive drugs for patients whose problems could, perhaps, be resolved if they simply ate less fat, lost weight and took exercise.

Q: Do you think that governments connive with the drug industry?

A: Yes, very much so. Governments are frightened of annoying drug companies because of their power and the money they bring into a country. To give a simple example: when they campaigned for victory in 1997, the British Labour party promised to investigate the usefulness of animal experiments. Many animal lovers voted for the Labour Party because of this. After the election, and under the influence of the drug companies, the Government lost all interest in stopping vivisection and did everything they could to make sure that the drug companies could do as many experiments as they liked. Even the most fervent enthusiasts for vivisection admit that they don't know which results they get are useful and which are not. If you don't know which tests are of any use they are all useless.

Q: What about government agencies which exist to protect patients and discipline doctors and drug companies?

A. I used to have more faith than I do now. I'm not sure whether I have become more suspicious or they have changed. Generally I don't have faith in any organisations which exist to protect patients. The problem is that there is too much movement between drug companies and these organisations. Scientists move from one to the other. And in many countries doctors and scientists work for drug companies and the advisory organisations.

Q: How could hospitals become better places for patients?

A: The ancient Egyptians and the Greeks had hospitals filled with music and flowers, etc. Modern hospitals are stressful, bug-ridden, bureaucratic and unfriendly. The patient is too often regarded as an inconvenience. Everyone working in hospital should remember that the most important person there is the patient. At least half of all administrators should be sacked and the money spent on taking better care of patients. Caring is an essential part of curing.

Q: What about accusations of doctors receiving money to research new drugs and then not publicising bad or inconvenient results?

A: I have for many years protested publicly about the way that drug companies will suppress inconvenient results. The drug companies should be severely punished for this.

Q: What is the main problem with medicines — the side effects they produce or their poor efficacy?

A: Drugs are often not as effective as drug companies say they are. But the big problem is side effects. I don't believe there is a single drug in the world which doesn't have side effects. If a patient takes a drug to save his life then side effects don't matter too much. But if the drug is being taken for some small problem then it is a tragedy if the drug kills him.

Q: Which drugs do you think are most wildly overprescribed?

A: Tranquillisers and anti-depressants have ruined many lives by being overprescribed. But the overuse of antibiotics is probably causing the biggest problems with the emergence of many resistant bugs. Anti-cancer drugs are largely a joke. The world would probably be a better and safer place without any of them. They are hugely profitable but I suspect they kill more people than they save.

Q: What about the growing trend for governments, drug companies and doctors to encourage self-medication?

A: All three encourage self-medication but for different reasons. Governments want people to buy their own drugs because it saves the government money. Drug companies want to sell drugs direct to patients because the profits are higher. And doctors encourage self-medication because it means less work for them. Self-medication is fine if patients know what they are taking and why. Unfortunately, the information available is often patchy, unreliable and inadequate. Patients overuse drugs and suffer nasty side effects as a result. If a patient taking a drug develops new symptoms then, by Coleman's 1st Law Of Medicine, the new symptoms are caused by the drug.

Q: Do medicines damage the human organism's defence mechanisms?

A: I strongly believe that the human body has sound defences against illness. I first wrote about this in my book *Bodypower* in 1983. Overuse of drugs damages these self-defence mechanisms and makes the individual more vulnerable.

Q: Sum up your attitude towards prescription drugs.

A: Drugs can save lives. But they can also kill. We need more doctors who understand the benefits and dangers more fully and more objectively.

Q: Do you think that medical researchers ever waste time and money?

A: Drug companies spend too much time and money looking for me-too drugs; new variations on profitable themes. They are, for example, constantly looking for new tranquillisers and anti-depressants because these are profitable. And they are constantly introducing new drugs which are promoted with great enthusiasm because they fit a marketing niche and then quietly withdrawn and forgotten a few years later. And remember that drug companies often create markets for their drugs by creating illnesses — as they have done so successfully for example with drugs for the menopause. If drug company executives really cared about people and about communities most would close their companies. Drug companies produce endless money-making variations of the same drugs, which do absolutely nothing for anyone except employees and shareholders.

Q: The incidence of psychological disease is increasing dramatically. Do you have any idea why?
A: There are huge profits to be made out of tranquillisers, sleeping tablets and anti-depressants. Most of the patients taking these drugs don't need them and don't benefit from them. The only people who really benefit are the drug companies. Doctors prescribe these drugs because handing out prescriptions is quicker and easier than investigating causes and offering proper advice.

Q: You say that doctors are not taught well. How should medical students be taught?
A: Students should be taught true holistic medicine. They should learn to see the patient as a person. And they should investigate all the causes of an illness (environment, immune system, stress etc.) before offering a solution. Students should be taught that

patients can benefit from a mixture of treatments including, where necessary, drugs, surgery and alternative medicine.

Q: Do you think that doctors are slow to accept new ideas?

A: Doctors have been very slow to recognise the importance of diet in health. There has been evidence for decades showing that meat causes cancer. If you eat lots of meat you are more likely to die of cancer. That's a fact. Doctors don't see this because they rarely read original research. They just read the leaflets handed out by the drug companies — which only mention drug therapies. And the medical journals, which make huge amounts of money from drug company advertising, don't deal with these issues either. I recently read about a doctor who was prescribing meat for his patients because he thought it would make them healthier. I reported him to the General Medical Council on the grounds that he was doing something that was dangerous to his patients but the General Medical Council wasn't interested, of course. The General Medical Council is far more concerned with defending the establishment than looking after patients' interests.

Q: What damage can medical check-ups cause to patients? Don't you think that medical check-ups can discover disease in early stages?

A: Check-ups are no more use than a single bank statement. If you had one bank statement a year it would give you a false view of your financial health. Medical check-ups produce a lot of false negatives and false positives and give people a false sense of security. It is much better to tell patients what problems to look out for — and to tell them of the significant warning signs that show impending problems.

Q: What damage can occur after taking vaccines?

A: Vaccines have caused (and cause) enormous problems. I have been a critic since the 1970s. They can damage the brain and the body. Their value is wildly overemphasised and their danger wildly underemphasised. The problem is that some vaccines do prevent the spread of diseases. But at high cost to individuals. Governments don't mind sacrificing individuals for the good of the community. I don't think doctors should do this. Anyone having a vaccination should make sure that their doctor signs a document taking responsibility if things go wrong (if patients did this, there would be far fewer vaccinations.) There has been much research showing the dangers of vaccines. But some of this research is suppressed because it is inconvenient. I first became aware of the dangers with the whooping cough vaccine. But I have grave doubts about all vaccines. My books contain more specific information.

Q: Don't you think vaccines have helped eradicate diseases such as polio? Isn't this a good argument in favour of vaccination? In poor regions diseases such as measles are very dangerous. Aren't vaccines a way to prevent many deaths?

A: If you accept that thousands of individuals will die or suffer great disabilities for the sake of the community then vaccines probably have a place. I think the price is too great. Many great claims are made for vaccines. But the claims are usually overdone. Many diseases were reducing in numbers long before vaccines were introduced. Better living conditions and antibiotics — not vaccines — are responsible. If you look at the graphs you will see that infectious diseases were falling before vaccines were introduced and that vaccines now kill or injure more people than they save.

Q: The world dreams of a vaccine against AIDS or cancer. Do you think it's a possibility?
A: No, There are much better ways to deal with the problems. Improving the immune system is the key.

Q: The risk of a hospital infection is high, but some diseases have to be treated inside hospital. How can a patient know whether the risk is worth it or not?
A: If their condition will kill them if they do not go into hospital then going to hospital is obviously essential. But I would try to keep out of hospital for things which did not threaten my life.

Q: Does the body have the power to cure diseases alone?
A: Definitely. I have written about this in books such as *Bodypower, Mindpower* and *Superbody.*

Q: Don't you accept that medical advances are responsible for increases in life expectation.
A: No. This is a myth put forward by drug companies and the medical establishment. Better living conditions are responsible for a reduction in infant mortality. And it is the reduction in infant mortality which has led to apparently greater life expectation. People who had survived childhood often lived to their 80's or 90's a century or two ago. There are more old people around today because populations have grown. And there are problems dealing with them because there is more chronic illness and because young families no longer have the time or money to look after their old.

Q: Do you think that the return of the old-fashioned family doctor could improve things?
A: Definitely. The real family doctor acts as the patient's interpreter and agent, helping to guide patients through every available form of diagnosis or treatment, explaining what is going on and providing support.

Sadly, real family doctors are now a rarity. The money is spent on unnecessary drugs and on administration instead.

Q; You have said that during some doctors' strikes the mortality rates decreased. Is that really the case?

A: Yes. Too many investigations and too much treatment causes many illnesses. In many instances the body can heal itself without medical help.

Q: What is the secret of a good doctor?

A: The doctor should listen, listen and listen. Very often a good doctor can learn more from talking and listening than from examining. High-tech medicine is all very well, but just listening is still crucial. And many doctors don't find the time to listen.

Q; Is being a vegetarian a good way to prevent disease?

A: Yes. There is no doubt about this. The scientific evidence is summarised in my book *Food for Thought* and on my website.

Q: Are you vegetarian?

A: Yes. I am vegetarian because I don't want to eat animals. But this is not why I recommend that readers follow a vegetarian diet. I believe that eating meat causes many diseases and that a vegetarian diet is much healthier. If I believed that meat was essential it would be my responsibility as an author to tell the truth — though I would still not eat meat myself.

Q: Were you given vaccines as a child?

A: I was given some vaccines as a child and, fortunately, I was one of the lucky ones: I survived them. But when I was a child we were given far fewer vaccines than children are given these days. The risks from most of the diseases for which vaccines are now given are slight. For example, measles does not kill many children. Vaccines are given for the economic benefit of the community rather than the health of the individual. If you approve of that then you can approve of vaccines. I consider it to be a fascist political attitude rather than a healing, humanitarian attitude.

We hope you found this book useful. If so we would be grateful if you would post a favourable review on Amazon.

Vernon Coleman is a qualified doctor and the author of over 100 books which have sold over two million hardback and paperback copies in the UK and been translated into 25 languages. His other medical books include 'Bodypower', 'Mindpower', 'Spiritpower', 'Superbody', 'How to Stop Your Doctor Killing You', 'Do Doctors and Nurses Kill More People than Cancer' and 'Food for Thought'. He has written more than a dozen novels, including 'Mrs Caldicot's Cabbage War' which was turned into an award winning movie. He is the author of the hugely popular Bilbury series of books. Many of his books are available as kindle books on Amazon. There is a list of his books on his author page on Amazon. For more information please see http://www.vernoncoleman.com/

Manufactured by Amazon.ca
Bolton, ON

14973575R00164